Stay healthy

Thanks for your support,

Remember, To live forever

Don't Die !!!

I met Dr. Williams in 2007 and was immediately impressed by his mild demeanor and good mannerisms. Little did I know at the time that he would become one of the most important people in my life. He has not only transformed his own body, but has helped hundreds of people like myself get in the best shape of their lives.

—MIKE BUTTE
Patient turned friend turned fan
President & CEO, Z-CO Development

Dr. Vernon Williams' book is the key to the Fountain of Youth and Anti-aging. He establishes the ability to synthesize the pharmacogenomics of patient-specific medicine with the latest scientific breakthroughs in anti-aging. This book is an invaluable tool and must-have reading for all.

—WELTHA CREASMAN, PhD-PharmD, MBA, BS PHARM, RPH

In *Grow Younger Like Me*, Dr. Williams takes us on a page-by-page journey as he demonstrates his strong passion to help his patients and readers. This incredible book is a must read for anyone interested in their health and happiness. It will be your guide to regain your vibrant, youthful past.

—DERRICK M. DeSILVA JR., MD
Chairman, Planning Committee
Age Management Medicine Group (AMMG)

The brightest physicians today realize that in order to age healthier and live to our fullest potential, no matter what our age, we must be pro-active in our health. Conventional medicine and disease management has failed us. I congratulate Dr. Vernon Williams on his new book *Grow Younger Like Me*. It allows readers to feel their best and avoid being part of our over-medicated society. I am honored that the BioTE Hormone Optimization Method is part of his five-step process.

—GARY DONOVITZ, MD
Founder and Medical Director, BioTE Medical

Dr. Williams isn't just an expert—he truly practices what he preaches! He combines first-hand knowledge and a unique understanding to create a system that can make you *feel and look younger*, almost instantly.

—PHILIP KUJAWSKI
Founder, WebToMed.com

Being in Dr. Williams' care for the last year has dramatically changed my well- being. I am a 44-year-old woman, but I honestly feel like I'm in my 20s. I feel blessed to have found him and his wonderful staff.

—ELIZABETH MARES
Patient

Most of us aspire to long life, and yet, what is longevity without quality? It would be prudent then to protect our health and vitality. I highly recommend Dr. Williams' book as a means of achieving this end. Consider it your "Health Bible" to keep you well from the top of your head to the soles of your feet.

—SYLVIA PETERSON, RPh

Dr. Williams is the epitome of how a doctor should be. Being versed in all aspects of health and wellness truly allows Dr. Williams to find the real underlying cause of the patients' concerns. He is the professional's professional!

—JASON ROBBINS
President of Men's Wellness Centers

Dr. Vernon Williams combines his brilliance in medicine with his own personal journey back to health to deliver a book that will change your life. Nothing beats a broad knowledge combined with a personal journey. Read this book; then live this book as a gift to yourself and to the people you love.

—CHARLES RUNELS, MD
Inventor of the O-Shot ® and Priapus Shot ® procedures

I have known Dr. Williams as both a colleague and "patient" for several years. He constantly strives to learn how to best care for his patients and has looked well beyond the scope of mainstream medicine and it's limitations. In this book, he has carefully crafted the synthesis of this knowledge. He is spot on!

—WILLIAM SHEA, MD

Between Dr. Williams discovering that my thyroid was not functioning properly, and the fact that my testosterone and estrogen levels were well below where they needed to be, *my life has completely changed.* POW! My marriage of 22 years has regained more than its original spark, my business is growing at an amazing rate, and I look and feel younger than I have in a very, very long time.

—TINA SMITH
Patient

Dr. Williams has managed to package a ton of information into a concise, readable, and understandable book. This information is vital if you want to reach and maintain optimal health throughout your life. If you start by implementing even just a few of the concepts in this book, you will feel and look younger.

—ELDRED B. TAYLOR, MD OB/GYN
Author of *Are Your Hormones Making You Sick*
and *The Stress Connection*

Dr. Williams was and is a blessing. I have so much more energy and I feel so much healthier and happy. Dr. Williams' ultimate goal is for all of his patients to look and feel great about themselves; he has only their best interests at heart.

—CYNTHIA WEAVER
Patient

Dr. Williams is a rare physician, indeed. He treats people not diseases or symptoms. He is one of the most compassionate and authentically dedicated professionals I have ever known.

—KATHY HESS-RENEAU, MA, LPC
Certified Professional & Recovery Coach,
Mediator, Motivational Speaker

Grow
YOUNGER
like ME

VERNON F. WILLIAMS, MD

Grow YOUNGER like ME

BE 29 AGAIN AND AGAIN

*How To
Look,
Feel, &
Function
Younger
Without
Stress*

Advantage®

Published by Advantage, Charleston, South Carolina.
Member of Advantage Media Group.

ADVANTAGE is a registered trademark and the Advantage colophon is a trademark of Advantage Media Group, Inc.

Printed in the United States of America.

ISBN: 978-1-59932-475-3
LCCN: 2014936126

This publication is designed to provide accurate and authoritative information in regard to the subject matter covered. It is sold with the understanding that the publisher is not engaged in rendering legal, accounting, or other professional services. If legal advice or other expert assistance is required, the services of a competent professional person should be sought.

Advantage Media Group is proud to be a part of the Tree Neutral® program. Tree Neutral offsets the number of trees consumed in the production and printing of this book by taking proactive steps such as planting trees in direct proportion to the number of trees used to print books. To learn more about Tree Neutral, please visit www.treeneutral.com. To learn more about Advantage's commitment to being a responsible steward of the environment, please visit www.advantagefamily.com/green

Advantage Media Group is a publisher of business, self-improvement, and professional development books and online learning. We help entrepreneurs, business leaders, and professionals share their Stories, Passion, and Knowledge to help others Learn & Grow. Do you have a manuscript or book idea that you would like us to consider for publishing? Please visit advantagefamily.com or call 1.866.775.1696.

Contents

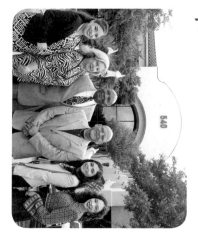

Free Aesthetics Consultations

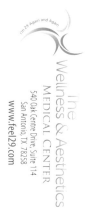

The
Wellness & Aesthetics
MEDICAL CENTER

540 Oak Centre Drive, Suite 114
San Antonio, TX 78258
www.feel29.com

I'm 29 Again and Again

Wellness / Age Management

- AGE MANAGEMENT MEDICINE/BHRT
- STRESS MANAGEMENT
- WEIGHT REDUCTION
- ENERGY MEDICINE
- CONCIERGE MEDICINE
- GENETIC TESTING
- IV NUTRITION
- PERSONAL CUSTOMIZED VITAMINS
- FOOD & ENVIRONMENTAL
- ALLERGY TESTING
- FIBROMYALGIA &
- CHRONIC FATIGUE SYNDROME
- NEUROTRANSMITTER TESTING
  & TREATMENT
- TESTOSTERONE & ESTROGEN PELLETS
- LYME DISEASE
- AUTO IMMUNE DISEASE/LEAKY GUT
- ADHD, PTSD, DEPRESSION
- INTEGRATIVE CANCER THERAPY
- PRP AND STEM CELL THERAPY
- HYPOTHYROID THERAPY

Sexual Health

- M SHOT (PRIAPUS, GAINS ENHANCEMENT/WAVE)
- O SHOT
- VAGINAL REJUVENATION
- NIPPLE REJUVENATION
- WOMEN'S SEXUAL DYSFUNCTION
- ERECTILE DYSFUNCTION (ED)
- PREMATURE EJACULATION (PE)

Aesthetics

- TICKLE LIPO BODY SCULPTURING
- LASER HAIR REDUCTION
- VAMPIRE FACE LIFT / VAMPIRE HAIR REGROW
- PHOTOFACIAL LASER TREATMENTS
- LASER ACNE TREATMENTS
- LASER SKIN TYTE/WRINKLE REDUCTION
- FACIAL FILLERS & MUSCLE RELAXATION
- MICRODERMABRASION/CHEMICAL PEELS
- FACIAL REJUVENATION with CELL
- AUGMENTATION (FAT+STEM CELLS + PRP)
- FACIAL REJUVENATION with YLIFT
- LASER REDUCTION OF SMOKERS LINES
- LASER LOWER EYELID TREATMENTS
- LASER HAIR REGROW
- SKIN CARE WITH GENETIC TESTING

www.Feel29.com • www.BecomeSexyAgain.com • www.GrowYoungerAgain.com • www.LookBeautifulAgain.com

(210) 495-8558 • 540 Oak Centre Drive, Suite 114 • San Antonio, TX 78258

Near North Central Baptist Hospital

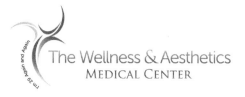
The Wellness & Aesthetics
MEDICAL CENTER

Introduction

WHAT WOULD YOU GIVE TO LOOK AND FEEL 29 AGAIN?

*I*f you're serious about reclaiming your youthful look and feeling, you've come to the right source. My name is Dr. Vernon Williams; I'm a physician and the author of this book. In my book, you'll learn the steps you can take, starting now, to improve your health, energy, happiness, function, looks, attitude, and lifestyle. My goal is nothing less than making you feel like your old, young self again—as I do.

Getting started on this journey begins with an accurate, honest assessment of where you are now. If, for instance, you wanted to go to New York City, you'd first need to know from where you're starting out, because the route to NYC from San Antonio is different than it is from Tokyo. In order to determine where you are now, we first need to understand how the medical system you're using works—or doesn't. Here's a checklist:

- What are your health care practitioners telling you?
- What are their beliefs (myths)?
- Where are they getting their information?
- What are their objectives?

- Are they trying to fix the root causes of your medical problems, or simply slapping Band-Aids on them?

Before we get started, I'd like to tell you a little about me, and my personal wellness journey. I was born in Trinidad & Tobago, and then moved to Harlem, New York City, where I met my parents for the first time at the age of 10. I graduated from Harvard University with a BA in biology, and then attended Albert Einstein Medical School. I did a General Surgery residency at Allegheny General Hospital and became a Flight Surgeon in the U.S. Air Force. Subsequently, I became an Emergency Medicine Physician prior to leaving the U.S. Air Force.

In 1992, I was diagnosed with a pituitary adenoma (prolactinoma). I gained 75 pounds and my breasts became a size D. For the first time, I was on the other side of the examination table; I was the patient, seeing firsthand how limited and ineffectual the medical response to my condition was. Rather than treating my underlying problem, my endocrinologist put a pharmaceutical band-aid on me. As far as he was concerned, it was just fine that I would be on medications for the rest of my life. He did not attempt to find the cause or fix the problem. My realization that this represented the prevailing attitude in modern medicine was the impetus that started me on the journey that's brought me to where I am today. Today, I look and feel younger than I did 15 years ago. My physio-age analysis indicates a composite score of 28 years.

In the chapters to come, I'll explain how I accomplished my own "medical miracle"—and how you can, too.

Now, let's start our journey toward growing younger, by exploring some of the most common, and damaging, medical myths.

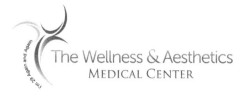
Chapter One

MEDICAL MYTHS

Most people, including a lot of medical professionals who ought to know better, believe a number of medical myths. In terms of your lifestyle, health choices, and medical treatments, belief in these myths can very well undermine your health, rather than support it. Let's look at and debunk some of the major medical myths commonly believed today.

MYTH #1: PERFORMANCE-ENHANCING DRUGS (PED) ARE BAD FOR YOU

According to Wikipedia, **performance-enhancing drugs** are substances used by people to improve their performance in the sports in which they engage. The term may also refer to drugs used by military personnel to enhance combat performance.

Although the phrase *performance-enhancing drugs* is typically used in reference to the kinds of anabolic steroids we associate with disgraced pro athletes, world anti-doping organizations apply the term far more broadly. Among the classes of drugs to which the phrase is usually applied are:

- *Painkillers* mask athletes' pain so they can continue to compete and perform when injured or sore. These increase blood pressure, causing the cells in the muscles to be better supplied with needed oxygen. Painkillers used by athletes range from ibuprophen to powerful prescription narcotics.

- *Lean mass drugs* are used to speed up the growth of lean body mass and muscle, or to reduce body fat. This class of drugs includes anabolic steroids and human growth hormone.

- *Stimulants* push the body and mind beyond their limits to perform at optimal level by increasing focus, energy, and aggression. Familiar stimulants include caffeine, amphetamine, and methamphetamine.

- *Sedatives* are sometimes used by athletes to overcome excessive nervousness, or in sports that require steady hands, such as target shooting. Common examples of these would be alcohol, marijuana, and valium.

- *Diuretics* cause the body to shed water, and are most often used by athletes who need to lose weight quickly in order to meet a weight class limit; for instance, boxers or wrestlers.

The decisions as to whether to include or exclude certain substances under the heading of performance-enhancing drugs (PED) is more than a little arbitrary. Anabolic steroids and human growth hormone are considered PED, but vitamins and supplements are not usually considered performance enhancers, though they clearly can impact an athlete's performance.

The definition of PEDs—"substances used by people to improve their performance in the sports in which they engage"—is quite flexible. Take as an example a woman getting ready to go out on a date, given that dating can arguably be defined as a competitive sport. She puts on her makeup (arguably a PED), and drinks a cup of coffee (another PED.) She probably puts on a relatively skimpy, sexy outfit (a sort of PED), and despite the cold outside, most likely goes out without a jacket to optimize the outfit's effectiveness. You could argue that, like a sport, dating is an enterprise in which success relates strongly to preparation. Under that rubric, applying for a job could also be classed as a competitive sport. In both cases, you optimize your resume and dress for success, and do your best to be as sharp as you possibly can be in your interview.

If there was a substance that made a trial lawyer intellectually optimal, that helped him to win all his cases, do you think he would go for it? If there were a drug that could make an older woman younger and more beautiful, would she be likely to take it? If an executive had been the top dog for a long time, but now saw his younger associate trying to take his job, would he take the PED that would make him feel more vigorous and competitive? I think it is very likely that the answer to all of these is a resounding "yes!" In the United States, we have freedom to choose what we wish to use to optimize our own performance, provided it does not harm another.

The term "survival of the fittest" describes a world in which only the strongest survive. In the animal kingdom, that is clearly true: it is kill or be killed. Man is just a civilized animal, even granted that, for the most part, we have modified the notion of survival of the fittest into a non-life-ending event. That said, there is still an element of competition in everything we do. To cherry-pick the things we do and decide that one thing qualifies as a PED, while another does not, seems morally questionable, if not in fact depraved.

My objective in this book is to show you how to optimize your body naturally, and how to enhance your performance using natural remedies. The most powerful enhancers are:

- Sleep

- Exercise

- Nutrition (vitamins, minerals, herbs, and enzymes)

- Optimizing your weight

- Detoxifying your body

- Optimizing your hormonal balance, using bio-identical hormones.

With these natural PEDs working for you, you will be more energized, lighter on your feet, mentally more alert, have less stress, and have younger, healthier skin. Like me, you can and will look and feel 29 again.

MYTH #2: STEM CELLS SHOULD BE AVOIDED

While the use of human embryonic stem cells has created considerable controversy, there is little doubt in the medical research world that they have tremendous potential to treat myriad diseases and health conditions, potentially including Alzheimer's and Parkinson's diseases, as well as applications in preventative medicine, cosmetic medicine, cancer, arthritis, degenerative disc disease, and spinal cord disease.

Stem cell research got a politicized setback because of the use of embryonic stem cells. It has made a comeback because of its undeniable medical potential. The prospect of their use figuring in curing most diseases, as well as their potential for use in regenerating organs, is too strong to deny. There is also promise in their use in preventative medicine and the cosmetic realm.

What kinds of potential are we talking about? In 2011, a group of scientists in Hong Kong and the United States suggested that research using stem cells might well lead to growing replacement parts for the human heart within the next five years. Texas Governor Rick Perry announced in 2011 that he had received an injection of his own stem cells during spinal fusion surgery. A company called Advanced Cell Technology has spent more than a decade working on treatments for eye disease that use embryonic stem cells.

And the good news for those who find the source of these cells ethically troublesome is that researchers are finding other sources, such as human body fat, to be even more promising as a supply of stem cells for regenerative therapies. Stem cells are being used to heal wounds, and back pain. A breakthrough in the treatment of diabetes mellitus is on the horizon, as adult stem cells have been induced to insulin-producing cells and/or islet clusters. Islet precursor cells exist within the pancreas and can be induced to differentiate into Beta cells.

How many people might potentially benefit from the research going on in the stem cells and regenerative medicine? The numbers are simply mind-boggling. Current medical challenges which might be addressed by regenerative technologies, include:

- Congestive Heart Failure (5 million U.S. patients)
- Osteoporosis (10 million U.S. patients)
- Alzheimer's Disease (5.5 million U.S. patients)
- Parkinson's Disease (5.5 million U.S. patients)
- Severe burns (0.3 million patients)
- Spinal Cord Injuries (0.25 million patients)
- Birth Defects (0.15 million)
- Diabetes Mellitus (24 million U.S. patients; 217 million world wide; Type I = 10–20% of total)

With more Texans opting to go to other countries and spending an inordinate amount of money on treatments unavailable to them in Texas, the Texas Medical Board voted to allow stem cell usage in Texas. Hopefully, this will open the door for the other states to allow the use of stem cells.

MYTH #3: CHOLESTEROL IS BAD FOR YOU

Cholesterol is a chemical compound that is naturally produced by the body. Structurally, it's a combination of lipid (fat) and steroid. Cholesterol is a building block for cell membranes and for hormones such as estrogen, progesterone, testosterone, DHEA, cortisol, pregnenolone, and corticosterone. The liver produces about 80 percent of the body's cholesterol, while the rest comes from our diet. The main sources of dietary cholesterol are meat, poultry, fish, and dairy products. Organic meats, such as liver, are especially high in cholesterol content, while foods of plant origin contain no cholesterol. After a meal, dietary cholesterol is absorbed from the intestine and stored in the liver. The liver is able to regulate cholesterol levels in the blood stream and can secrete cholesterol if the body needs it.

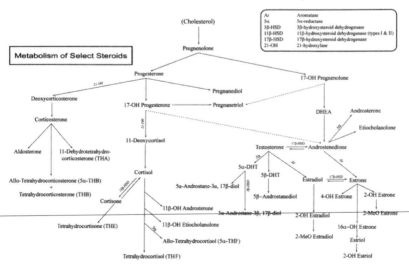

We hear a lot about the dangers of cholesterol, but very little about what it actually does for us in the body. What are the functions of cholesterol?

Cholesterol performs many important functions within our bodies:

- Cholesterol provides stability to cell membranes to enable them to selectively regulate vital substances needed for our survival to enter and exit the cell.

- Cholesterol maintains the structure of vessels.

- Overly low cholesterol levels will suppress your immune system, making you susceptible to illnesses and diseases.

- Cholesterol is one of the body's natural cancer protectors.

- Cholesterol produces hormones, which assist with healing your body from injury or infections.

- Cholesterol acts as an insulator around nerves and protects your nervous system from diseases.

- Cholesterol is a major participant in the production of Vitamin D. Vitamin D is a valuable nutrient for strong bones, a robust immune and nervous system, procreation, production of insulin and creation of energy from absorbed or ingested minerals.

- Cholesterol is imperative for your brain to function.

- Cholesterol is influential on your memory capacity.

- Cholesterol plays a role in hormones reaching your brain.

- Serotonin receptors in the brain need cholesterol to function properly. Serotonin is an important neurotransmitter. Low levels of serotonin can cause depression, anxiety, mood swings, temperature regulation difficulties, loss of libido and appetite, and sleep disorders.

- Cholesterol produces testosterone, estrogen, and progesterone. Lowering of cholesterol can result in loss of sexual drive, lethargy, fatigue, hot flashes, menstrual irregularities, pregnancy miscarriages, and bone mineral density deficiency.

- Cholesterol is important to steroid hormone production. There are five classes of steroid hormones: (1) androgens, which affect maturation and function of secondary sex organs for male sexual determination; (2) estrogens; (3) progesterone; (4) mineralocorticoids, which are responsible for maintaining salt and water balance; and (5) glucocorticoids, which increase stress resistance.

- A healthy level of cholesterol is required for digestion. Cholesterol forms bile in the liver. Bile aids in absorption of the food we consume. A lack of bile will induce digestive symptoms, such as diarrhea.

- Cholesterol strengthens our intestinal walls.

- The insulin hormone, which is related to your blood sugar levels, is made from cholesterol.

- Lower-than-normal cholesterol levels may accelerate signs of aging. As a result, age-related diseases may manifest themselves at an earlier age. A finding published in the *American Journal of Medicine* over 20 years ago showed that risks for an early death increased if cholesterol levels are too low.

- Studies reveal there may be an association between Parkinson's disease and cholesterol levels.

- People with kidney dysfunction are at an increased risk if their cholesterol levels are lowered.

- The body makes 80 percent of its cholesterol; only 20 percent comes through our diet.

The big take-away here is that cholesterol is naturally formed in the body. It is imperative for our survival. To attempt to reduce your cholesterol level to such a degree that it cannot carry out its purposes may be dangerous to your health and lead to early death.

Cell membranes require cholesterol in order to function properly. Cholesterol maintains the correct fluidity of the cell membrane at different temperatures. Cholesterol protects the permeability of the cell membrane. The brain contains a large amount of cholesterol compared to other organs in the body. The cholesterol in the brain is generally found in the myelin sheaths and protects the cells and helps to ensure electrical impulses occur within this organ. The liver uses cholesterol to synthesize bile, an essential enzyme in digestion. Bile is useful in the breakdown and digestion of dietary fats. Synthesizing vitamin D from sunlight also requires cholesterol. Vitamin D is needed for bone health and calcium absorption. We could not survive without cholesterol.

Low-density lipoprotein (LDL) is often called "bad" cholesterol. It delivers cholesterol to the cells. High-density lipoprotein (HDL) is often called "good" cholesterol. It removes cholesterol from the bloodstream. You need both—and, clearly, the "bad" label is a slander on such an essential thing.

That said, like everything in life, too much of a good thing is just as bad as too little. Yes, too much cholesterol can cause plaque buildup. You can also drown with too much water. Cholesterol levels that are too low can cause serious complications, including death.

MYTH #4: CANCER IS CURED BY CHEMOTHERAPY

"Most cancer patients in this country die of chemotherapy. Chemotherapy does not eliminate breast, colon, or lung cancers. This fact has been documented for over a decade, yet doctors still use chemotherapy for these tumors." Allen Levin, MD, UCSF.

According to Ralph Moss in his book *Questioning Chemotherapy*, in a surprisingly high number of surveys, chemotherapists have responded that they would neither recommend chemotherapy for their families nor would they use it themselves. One of their advisors, Dr. Dan Harper, reported about an unpublished cohort study in which it was revealed that only 9 percent of oncologists would take chemotherapy for their cancers. Knowing that, if you found yourself faced with a cancer diagnosis, might you reconsider your options for treatment?

Now consider this: When you are diagnosed with cancer, you are suddenly worth $300,000 to the cancer industry. And yes, I said "industry."

"Despite widespread use of chemotherapies, breast cancer mortality has not changed in the last 70 years." Thomas Dao, MD.

A treatment stops being therapeutic when it does more harm than good, and there's mounting evidence that chemotherapy may do exactly that. Irwin Bross, a biostatistician for the National Cancer Institute, discovered that many cancers that are benign will not metastasize until they are hit with chemotherapy. He's found that many people who've been diagnosed with metastatic cancer did not have metastatic cancer until they got their chemotherapy.

For many cancers, chemotherapy just does not improve your survival rate. Some of these are colorectal, gastric, pancreatic, bladder, breast, ovarian, cervical, and *corpus uteri*, head and neck.

....

From the University of Iowa website March 31, 2007

Patients and caregivers shall be taught safe, proper handling and disposal of waste generated during continuous infusions of chemotherapy.

The following procedures should be implemented immediately if a chemotherapy leak or spill should occur:

1. Put on a pair of disposable latex gloves.

2. If chemo has spilled on clothing, remove immediately and take a shower, scrubbing the exposed skin with soap and water. Watch for redness, blistering, or a burning sensation. Contact your nurse to report the spill. She will give you further instructions, if necessary.

3. Remove any and all sharp objects, placing them into your sharps container or any can with a lid, such as a coffee can.

4. Soak up the spill with an absorbent disposable material, such as paper towels.

5. Disinfect the spill area with soap and water or a household cleaner such as window cleaner, 409, alcohol, bleach, or liquid carpet cleaner.

6. Put the absorbent material and the gloves into chemotherapy waste container or garbage bag and carefully mark it. The pharmacy personnel will pick it up later.

7. If a spill occurs on a patient's or caregiver's clothing or sheets, these articles should be washed separately from regular laundry in hot water.

8. If a spill occurs on unprotected furniture, the area should be scrubbed with soap and water and rinsed with clean water while wearing protective chemo safety gloves.

9. Patients and caregivers should be taught to use care when handling vomitus or excretions of the patient for 48 hours post treatment and to use good hand-washing technique.

If hazmat-level precautions are required to handle chemotherapy spills, why would you want these chemicals in your body? Why would you consider using radiation to nuke all your cells (unaffected and affected) in order to fight cancer?

Dr. Hardin Jones, professor of medical physics and physiology at the University of California, Berkeley, told an American Cancer Society panel:

My studies have proven conclusively that untreated cancer victims actually live up to four times longer than treated individuals. For a typical type of cancer, people who refused treatment lived for an average of 12.5 years. Those who accepted surgery or other kinds of treatment [chemotherapy, radiation, cobalt] lived an average of only three years...I attribute this to the traumatic effect of surgery on the body's natural defense mechanism. The body has a natural defense against every type of cancer.

Reading this, you might reasonably ask why previous studies of chemotherapy outcomes have not sounded a warning about the perils of this approach for patient health. The reason is simple: If a person dies during a chemotherapy study, that information is NOT included in the write-up, because the patient did NOT complete the study.

If you're facing a cancer diagnosis, and considering your treatment options, please consider this: There are, in fact, alternate approaches that work *with* the body rather than by poisoning it with chemicals or radiation. One such natural approach to fighting cancer is to starve the cancer cells while strengthening your natural killer cells. This can be accomplished by getting rid of cancer's favorite food (sugar) and strengthening your other cells with good healthy nutrition.

MYTH #5: IT'S OKAY TO EAT SUGAR IF YOU HAVE CANCER

Eating sugar is definitely NOT okay if you're a cancer patient, because elevated sugars cause a proliferation and the metastasis of cancer. There is a 40 percent higher risk of diabetic patients dying from cancer. Lack of exercise, obesity, and sugar increases the risk for most cancers. In over 80 percent of dietary studies, fruits and vegetables consumption provided significant protection against cancer, and there's a significant body of research to prove it:

- Approximately 200 studies looked at the relationship of fruit/vegetable intake and cancers (lung, colon, breast, esophagus, oral, stomach, bladder, pancreas, and ovarian cancers). Low fruit and vegetable intake increased risk of cancers two-fold.

- Meta-analysis of breast cancer risk and diet was conducted using data from 26 published studies from 1982 to 1997. Analysis confirms association between intake of vegetables and fruits and reduced risk for breast cancer. Risk reduced in high-intake groups. Vegetables *reduce risk* for breast cancer.

- Significant protection found: Lung: 24 of 25 studies. Oral, esophagus: 28 of 29 studies (mainly fruits). Pancreas, stomach: 26 of 30 studies (mainly vegetables). Colorectal, bladder: 23 of 38 studies. Cervix, ovary, endometrium: 11 of 13 studies.

- Review of 206 human cancer studies and 22 animal studies showed that the most important dietary factors in reducing cancer development were fruit and vegetables. Cancer rates were reduced 50 percent in people who ate mainly fruits and vegetables.

- High fruit/vegetable intake is associated with a 20–50 percent lower risk of cancer. Low fruit/vegetable intake is associated with a significant higher risk of cancers (at least 2-fold). *The World Research Cancer Fund Report* is a compelling summary in favor of healthy whole food in regard to lower cancer risk.

The fact is, everyone has cancer. We have over 100 trillion cells in our body. Every day, thousands mutate into cancer cells. Most of these do not progress to cancer. Our strong immune system destroys the mutated cells before they can spread. **To fight cancer, we need to starve the mutated cells by taking away their favorite food (sugar) and strengthen our immune systems.** (Unfortunately, that preventative approach is very inexpensive and would not net the American Cancer Society the huge profits they desire.)

MYTH #6: VACCINATIONS DO NOT CAUSE DIABETES

Diabetes is a major health problem in the United States, and the number of diabetics is increasing every year. In 1947, there were an estimated 600,000 cases of diabetes in the United States. Adult onset (controlled by diet and exercise) makes up 85–90 percent of diabetics. The other 10–15 percent requires daily injections of insulin. Even though the U.S. population has approximately doubled since the 1940s, the number of diabetics has risen more than 20 times in the same time span. In 1976, Henry Bearn wrote: "It is perhaps not generally appreciated that in the United States diabetes, or at least the recognition of the disease, has increased about 300 percent over the last fifteen years. It is the second leading cause of blindness, and the third cause of death. In 1950 there were 1.2 million diabetics in the United States."

According to the *National Diabetic Fact Sheet* (released 01/26/2011), there were 25.8 million diabetics in the United States, 7 million of whom are undiagnosed and 79 million who are prediabetic. That's a 21,000 percent increase in the past 60 years. The American Diabetes Association (ADA) released new research on March 6, 2013, estimating the total costs of diagnosed diabetes have risen to $245 billion in 2012 from $174 billion in 2007. The number of diabetics in the United States is expected to double to over 53 million by 2025.

Diabetes is a direct cause of heart disease, stroke, peripheral vascular disease, renal failure, blindness, hypertension, and death. With an estimated total health bill in the United States of almost $3 trillion per year, the annual bill for the care and treatment of diabetics is over $245 billion.

Diabetes is related to the pancreas. In 1922, Canadians Frederick Banting and Charles H. Best discovered that insulin was the culprit in diabetes onset as the beta cells of the pancreas stop performing their function. In 1976, Alexander Bearn wrote, "Diabetes appears to be one of those diseases in which susceptibility may be inherited but where environmental factors may lead to the onset of disease and illness." Viral infection, childhood vaccinations, and the presence of an autoimmune process have been recognized as possible causes for diabetes. The epidemic of autoimmune disease in the United States started in the 1950s correlates with the rise of diabetes.

Several of the vaccines administered for childhood diseases have been implicated in the cause of diabetes. The vaccine for pertussis (whooping cough), which is part of the DPT shot (diphtheria, pertussis, tetanus) given to all children, includes "pertussis toxin," a toxin secreted by the microbe, which causes whooping cough (the Bordetella pertussis). This toxin, which has been described as one of the most virulent poisons known to science, has a variety of effects on the body. Pertussis toxin affects the "islets of Langerhans," which are the insulin-secreting parts of the pancreas. Pertussis vaccine has been known in animal experiments to stimulate over-production of insulin by the pancreas, followed by exhaustion and destruction of the "islets," with consequent under-production of insulin. This leads to hypoglycemia and, ultimately, to diabetes.

As early as 1949, physicians called attention to low blood glucose in children who had severe reactions to the pertussis vaccine. In 1970, Margaret Pittman wrote, "The infant whose blood sugar level is influenced by food intake may be especially vulnerable to vaccine-induced hypoglycemia...the vaccine induces hypoglycemia in mice and rabbits."

In 1977, Gordon Stewart stated, "More than any other vaccine in common use, pertussis vaccine is known pharmacologically to provoke...hypoglycemia, due to increased production of insulin." Two Dutch researchers, Hannik and Cohen, observed in 1978, "Infants who show serious reactions following pertussis vaccination suffer from a failure to maintain glucose homeostasis." And two German researchers, Hennessen and Quast, found in 1979 that 59 out of 149 children who manifested adverse reactions to the pertussis vaccine developed symptoms of hypoglycemia.

The MMR (measles, mumps, rubella) vaccine has also been implicated as a cause of Type-I diabetes. Of the three vaccines making up the MMR shot, the rubella component is the major culprit. Rubella (German measles), like mumps, is known to be a cause of diabetes, and the action of the vaccine resembles that of the disease. If the disease can cause diabetes, so can the vaccine. In 1978, Margaret Menser said: "Since 1968 there has been increasing interest in the possibility that viral infection may play a part in the etiology of diabetes mellitus in man... [But] only one virus consistently produces diabetes in man—the congenitally acquired rubella virus." "Congenital rubella syndrome" is the name given to the group of impairments and disabilities often seen in babies whose mothers become infected with rubella during pregnancy. These impairments include: heart disease, mental retardation, deafness, and blindness.

In 1986, E. J. Rayfield and colleagues wrote: "The congenital rubella syndrome provides the best documentation in humans that a viral infection is associated with the subsequent development of insulin-dependent [Type-I] diabetes mellitus." In the 1960s and 1970s, researchers came to realize that the effect of the rubella virus does not end at the moment of birth, but that it remains in the organism of the baby and continues to exert its influence for many years thereafter. Especially to be noted is the fact that up to 20 percent of these individuals later come down with Type-I diabetes. This may take from five to 20 years to develop, indicating that the rubella virus remains active in the organism for all that time.

In 1989, Numazaki and colleagues infected laboratory cultures of human pancreatic islet cells with rubella virus. They found that these infected cells produced much lower levels of insulin and concluded, "these results suggest that rubella virus can infect human pancreatic islet cells and that such infection may lead to significant reductions in levels of secreted insulin."

In 1982, P. K. Coyle and colleagues demonstrated that "rubella-specific immune complex formation is frequent after vaccination and could be demonstrated in two-thirds of an unselected group of vaccinates for as long as eight months after vaccination." In fact, the virus has been found to persist in the body of the vaccinated person for as long as seven years after vaccination. This is not surprising, given that in congenital rubella syndrome the virus can persist for at least 20 years and, probably, for a lifetime.

E. J. Mayfield and colleagues wrote: "The mechanism of virus-induced diabetes is not known. Viruses associated with diabetes in animals may cause disease by (1) directly lysing [i.e., dissolving] the beta-cells; (2) triggering an autoimmune response; or (3) specifically impairing the secretory process of beta-cells through a persistent infection." He concluded that the second option was the most probable one: the generation of an autoimmune state in which the body, as it were, becomes allergic to itself or to a part of itself.

The rubella vaccine can also cause an allergic reaction. A Canadian survey in 1987 found "allergic reactions" in 30 children who reacted adversely to the MMR vaccine. Diabetes after a rubella vaccination probably represents a combined effect: the virus attacks the islet cells of the pancreas in an organism, which has already been weakened by an autoimmune reaction to the same virus. A study of haemophilus influenzae B (Hib) vaccine in 114,000 Finnish children found that those who received four doses of the vaccine had a higher incidence of Type-I diabetes than did those who received only one dose. According to J. Barthelow Classen, MD, a hepatitis B vaccination program in New Zealand that commenced in 1988 led to a 60 percent increase in Type-I diabetes in the recipients. In the under-20 age group, the incidence of Type-I diabetes prior to the vaccination campaign (i.e., from 1982–1991) was 18.2/100,000 person years. Classen's data have led the National Institute of Allergy and Infectious Diseases to request the Swedish health authorities to investigate the possible connection between the pertussis vaccine and Type-I diabetes. In Classen's view, the Hepatitis B vaccine and other vaccines can induce Type-I diabetes through the release of interferons, since interferons have already been implicated as causing autoimmunity, including Type-I diabetes. Classen also observes that the package inserts for the various hepatitis B vaccines on the market notes that they cause several autoimmune diseases, and the FDA itself has recognized that they can cause alopecia (baldness) of autoimmune origin.

MYTH #7: SYNTHETIC DRUGS ARE THE SAME AS NATURAL DRUGS

Natural drugs cannot be patented—and that's a problem for drug companies, who count on those patents to bring in big bucks. As a result, there is minimal return on investment on natural remedies. Drug companies would rather take a natural remedy and create a synthetic (a compound resembling the original but not identical), which can then be patented as a new compound (one that never existed since the world was formed) in order for the drug company to have all the rights and money associated with that drug for the next 20 years. Yet, the fact is that 80 percent of synthetic drugs are derived from a known natural remedy.

Your best hope for disease prevention is already in you, programmed into you, in fact. Your DNA (23 chromosomes from Mom and 23 from Dad) has all the information that has accumulated from all your ancestors since the dawn of time. If your ancestors survived the bubonic plague in 2100 B.C., your DNA (like a computer) will have memory of how it killed the deadly virus. Therefore, if the bubonic plague were to strike again, you would most likely survive. Your body knows how to handle natural drugs. Your liver knows how to break down the drugs because it has all the enzymes, minerals, and cofactors required to do it.

On the other hand, when you ingest a synthetic drug for the first time, your body takes notice. It says, *What is this? Is this good or bad? What is it for? How do I destroy it?* The immune system is activated and ready to attack it. The synthetic drug lands on the cells and tries to do what the natural chemical would do. The only problem is that the synthetic drug effect on the cell may be different than the natural compound. This can cause over- or under-stimulation of the cell. In the case of synthetic estrogens, for one instance, overstimulation of breast tissue leads to breast cancer.

The drug companies know this, of course. It takes a drug company about 10 years and $1 billion to make a new synthetic drug. That is $500 million for the process (laboratory, testing, clinical trials, FDA approval) and $500 million for the advertising. Let's say that after six years and $400 million spent on the new drug, the clinical trials show a lot of side effects. What is the drug company to do? The investment they've made in this drug means that it is ***too big to fail***—so the drug company hides the data. If the pill was going to cost $17, the drug company ups the cost to $20 and puts $3 per pill into the kitty for the future lawsuits that will come when those side effects start showing themselves.

To get doctors to order the drugs for patients, the drug company forces the doctor to listen to them. They advertise to the patients, telling them to ask their doctor for the synthetic drug. The doctor, not wanting to sound uninformed, accepts the drug representative's pitch with open ears. He looks at the favorable research data. As patients request the drug, the physician eagerly prescribes it. The patient gives him props for being so well informed. Years later, when all the side effects manifest themselves, the FDA pulls the drug from the market. The FDA gets praise for their actions (remember they approved the drug in the first place). The class action lawsuit is settled by the law firm, which makes millions. The clients get pennies. The drug company pays from their extra kitty and pockets all the other billions of revenue. The patients are left with their side effects. Countless numbers die from the drug that was supposed to heal them.

There have been more than 500 drugs that the FDA has initially approved and later pulled from the market. How much suffering and how many deaths have resulted from those drugs is impossible to quantify. If one patient dies from a physician's malpractice, that physician goes under intense scrutiny and his license could be pulled. The FDA has caused untold pain, suffering, and deaths—yet no scrutiny. You hear from patients, "I won't take it if it is not FDA approved". Natural remedies usually do not get FDA approval, because they cannot be patented. Therefore, it is cost prohibitive for a company to seek FDA approval if they cannot patent it.

MYTH #8: PHYSICIANS CURE PATIENTS

In medicine today, physicians do not cure patients. We (physicians) merely stick band-aids on our patients. If a patient has depression at age 15, hypothyroidism at 18, and hypertension at 20, the patient will be on medication for the rest of his or her life. Additionally, the patient will be on multiple medications until death. The drug companies, whose sole purpose is to sell drugs, have no incentive to get you off your medications. Physicians get most of their CMEs (continuing medical educations) from the drug companies. They are indoctrinated into the world of the drug companies. Natural cures are ignored, even though as we've said earlier, most synthetic drugs are based on natural remedies. Unlike synthetic drugs, natural cures are inexpensive and do not provide profit to the drug companies; therefore, most physicians are unaware of them. For the physician, it's simpler to write a prescription than to search for an alternate, actual cure. To search for the cure requires precious time from the physician, additional payments from the insurance companies (testing, additional doctor visits), and less profit to the drug companies.

Most patients have been brainwashed into thinking they are not sick, that as long as their medical condition is controlled by their prescription, they do not have a medical problem. But medications are a cover-up, not a cure. While they may control symptoms, they don't attack the underlying condition that created them. In my practice, I've stopped asking if my patient has any medical conditions. Rather, I ask them what medications they take.

MYTH #9: ANTACIDS AND H2 BLOCKERS ARE GOOD FOR YOU

Zantac, Pepcid, Tagamet, antacids, and other H2 blockers so commonly used to treat acid reflux and upset stomach are *not* good for you, despite some of them claiming to be "calcium-rich." They prevent the stomach from performing its natural and necessary functions. The two primary responsibilities of the stomach are to break down protein and to sterilize foods, both of which require strong acid. When you decrease the acidity of the stomach, you prevent it from functioning.

The stomach only secretes acid if food is in it. With a strong stomach acid, protein is digested within an hour of consumption. The acid secretion then ceases. With weakened stomach acid, which is the result of taking an antacid or H2 blocker, food remains in the stomach upward of five hours. Therefore, weak acid secretion continues for up to five hours. Additionally, the weakened acid does not kill all the pathogens and pesticides on the foods. Then, these pathogens get into the intestines and disrupt its normal flora. This leads to intestinal inflammation, leaky gut, food sensitivities, allergies, and autoimmune diseases. Once again, we would rather place a band-aid on the problem than fix the problem.

Now that we've shot down some commonly held health myths, let's look at the route that will take us to our goal of growing younger.

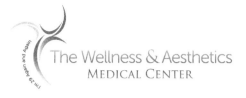

Chapter Two

GET WITH THE PROGRAM

My Five Steps Wellness Program is designed to help you to shave years off of your physical age and allow you to enjoy a veritable second youth. At the Wellness and Aesthetics Medical Center, we have been making people younger for the past three and a half years. It started with me: All the procedures we use start with either my personal experience or that of my office manager Mary's personal experience. I have been "29 again" for years.

My Five Steps wellness program is designed to optimize your body's systems and slow or reverse your biological age. These steps consist of **body sculpting, whole body detoxification, weight reduction, bio-identical hormone optimization, and customized vitamin and nutrition.** The five-step program is designed for everyone, but not everyone will need all five steps.

WHAT THE FIVE-STEP PROGRAM CAN DO FOR YOU

Here is what the five-step program can do for you:

- Reduce your weight
- Reduce your body fat
- Create a more desirable figure

- Optimize your hormones
- Reduce your stress
- Increase your sex drive
- Improve your metabolism
- Cleanse your body of unwanted toxins, bacteria, viruses, and funguses
- Decrease your blood pressure
- Improve your sleep pattern
- Improve your skin tone
- Increase your energy level
- Decrease your pain level
- Decrease your inflammation
- Decrease gastrointestinal discomforts
- Decrease your chances of getting coronary artery diseases, stroke, diabetes, or cancer
- Decreased your risks of other illness
- Improve your immune function

Now, let's have a look at the Five Steps themselves.

STEP 1. BODY SCULPTING

Liposuction has been around for a while, but recent innovations in technology and techniques have made it safer and easier than ever. PureLipo™ is an innovative, minimally invasive technique that sculpts and contours your body into a more sleek and desirable form by removing unwanted areas of excess fat from between the skin and muscle using a small tube or cannula. The PureLipo™ Body Sculpting technique provides significant advantages over traditional liposuction. PureLipo™ is better, safer, and more effective than traditional liposuction because it doesn't require general anesthesia, doesn't create tunnels through the fat, doesn't cause excessive fat removal, and does not generate dimpling of the skin, creating ridges and damaging the deep dermis.

The PureLipo™ procedure uses the **tumescent technique**. This technique involves the injection of small volumes of anesthetic fluid just underneath the skin where the fat (cells) lay. The anesthetic fluid makes the area swollen, firm, and numb. The fat cells are broken up and mixed with the fluid. The technique eliminates problems caused by general anesthesia and helps reduce the bleeding associated with traditional surgery. The tumescent technique makes the procedure harmless and less painful, with minimal post-procedural recovery time and superior cosmetic results.

After the procedure, you will be swollen and will experience drainage of the tumescent fluid, but most patients return to regular activities within 48 hours of treatment. You can expect to see results within 10 days. Weekly synergy (40 min. body massages) treatments for the next 10 weeks further help with the re-contouring of your body, and the reduction of swelling, weight, and cellulite. You will see significant total body sculpting within those 10 weeks and can expect to see the final results within six months.

Some of the most common body areas treated include: abdomen, inner and outer thighs, waist, back or flank area, upper arms, buttocks, breasts, face, and neck, although virtually any area can be treated. Fat cells that are removed by PureLipo™ do not grow back. As long as you do not gain excessive weight, the shape and contour is permanent.

Visit http://www.twaamc.com to see before and after photos.

STEP 2. WHOLE BODY DETOXIFICATION

The process of detoxification is ridding your body of toxins and restoring it to optimum health and vitality. We are always detoxing. When we breathe, we are removing harmful carbon dioxide. We are detoxing when we have a bowel movement or urinate. When we shower or perspire, we detox the skin. Brushing your mouth detoxifies it. Unfortunately, the world is producing g toxic chemicals at an alarming rate. Our body's tremendous ability to detoxify is being overwhelmed. As a result, toxins are being stored in our fat cells on a daily basis. Some of these toxins have half-lives of 30, 40, or even 50 years. We use IV Therapy to do Chelation to remove toxic metals from our patients. We also use IV Glutathione (the most powerful detoxifier in the body) to help detox the body.

Some of the benefits of detoxification include:

- Weight reduction
- Increased energy / vitality
- Better, more efficient digestion
- Decreased bloating, heartburn
- Younger, healthier skin
- Shinier, thicker hair
- Better sleep, decreased stress
- Sharper thinking and better memory
- Decreased pain

STEP 3. WEIGHT REDUCTION

Our approach to weight reduction goes above and beyond the usual "eat less and exercise more" prescription, with an approach that targets not only what you eat, but how those foods are metabolized. The key components in the design of our weight loss program are Glycemic Index, and the use of HCG, a hormonal weight loss supplement.

What is the "Glycemic Index"?

A low glycemic index and load diet can help you lose weight and to improve Type 2 diabetes. The glycemic index (GI) is a numerical system of measuring how much of a rise in circulating blood sugar a nutrient triggers—the higher the number, the greater the blood sugar response. A low GI food will cause a small rise, while a high GI food will trigger a dramatic spike.

Not all nutrients have the same effects on the body. After we eat foods that contain carbohydrates, for instance, our blood glucose level rises with a speed called "glycemic response." Glycemic response is influenced by the amount and the types of food we eat, and how the food is processed or prepared. When we eat a boiled potato, glucose levels spike in milliseconds. With legumes or fruits and vegetables, the levels go up in about 30 minutes. In general, a lower glycemic response means a better quality of food. Foods that have lower Glycemic response (glycemic index) cause only small fluctuations in blood sugar levels. This leads to lower insulin levels, which reduce the risk of coronary heart disease and diabetes. It also helps you to maintain a healthy weight.

The glycemic load (GL) is a relatively new way to assess the impact of carbohydrate consumption. It takes the glycemic index into account, but gives a better picture than does glycemic index alone. A GI value tells you only how rapidly a particular carbohydrate turns into sugar. It doesn't tell you how much of that carbohydrate is in a serving of a particular food. You need to know both things to understand a food's effect on blood sugar. The carbohydrate in watermelon, for example, has a high GI. But there isn't a lot of it, so watermelon's glycemic load is relatively low. A GL of 20 or more is high, a GL of 11 to 19 inclusive is medium, and a GL of 10 or less is low. Eating foods with GI less than 50 and GL less than 10 would ensure weight loss and reduction in Type 2 diabetes.

What is HCG?

HCG is a natural hormone that is safe and effective. If combined with a very low calorie diet (500 calories a day) and used under a doctor's supervision, you can quickly shed pounds, feel fine, maintain energy, and reduce your appetite all at the same time. HCG suppresses your appetite by resetting your hypothalamus, and releases 1,500-4,000 calories from stored fat per day. It increases your energy while burning fat. Most people using it lose an average of .5 to 1 pound per day. It is safe for both men and women.

Dr. A.T.W. Simeon created the HCG Diet in the 1950s. Dr. Simeon had a large clinic in Rome, Italy. People from around the world would come to go on his diet and lose weight. His diet and his work are discussed in his book *Pounds and Inches*. How does it work? HCG forces your body to utilize its stored fat, thus causing you to lose weight rather rapidly. HCG is a prescription drug that must be prescribed by a physician to be legal. It is unwise to purchase it off the Internet.

In order to do the program in a safe and healthy way, you should start by meeting with a physician who is knowledgeable about HCG, who can follow and monitor you regularly, who can write a prescription for HCG, and who follows an HCG Diet program protocol that works. Numerous changes occur within your body when you eat only 500 calories a day. You need to know the correct types of foods that you can eat and the correct way to do the program. Proper monitoring to prevent potential problems associated with a low calorie diet is essential for ensuring your safety.

STEP 4. BIO-IDENTICAL HORMONE OPTIMIZATION

Age Management medicine is a way to slow down the aging process and optimize your body's health. There are many who believe that you get older because your hormone levels decline. Your hormone levels are at their peak between 25 and 35 years old. After this point, your hormone levels begin to drop. Bio-identical Hormone Replacement Therapy (BHRT) is a technique used to treat hormone deficiencies that arise as we age. Bio-identical hormones are those that are molecularly identical to the hormones that are produced in the body. These hormones are used to treat pre- and post-menopausal and andropausal symptoms. Bio-identical hormones are customized to each individual's needs and deficiencies. They are identical to those your body produces, and therefore free of any side effects. In order for this to work, the hormones you take have to be personalized for your body chemistry, to increase your own specific, unique, biological functions and improve your individual quality of life. This is impossible with commercially produced synthetic hormones.

Bio-identical hormones are much different from synthetic hormone replacement in that bio-identical hormones are metabolized, stored, and converted into other hormones naturally. Bio-identical hormones are of the exact same chemical structure as those produced by your body. Synthetic hormones are generic and the same hormone will affect every person differently. BHRT is derived from plants instead of animals and therefore no animal byproducts or horse urine is used.

Synthetic hormones are not identical to those in the human body. Most are produced from animals and have different chemical structures and functions than that of human hormones. These hormones produce side effects. After the synthetic hormone is absorbed and used, it produces a byproduct that is significantly different from those produced from human hormones. These byproducts could be needed for other functions in your body or could just be waste. In the synthetic hormone, the byproduct might not have the right characteristics needed for these pathways and could potentially be harmful.

In contrast, bio-identical hormones are natural and are metabolized normally, and as stated earlier, will produce virtually **NO** side effects. Synthetic hormones can often be quite strong and may produce unbearable side effects.

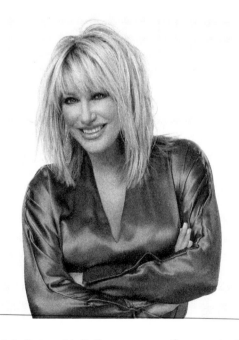

As a member of the Forever Health Network, whose National Spokesperson is Suzanne Somers, I'm involved with a consortium of physicians dedicated and trained in Bio-identical Hormone Replacement which is life changing. Forever Health and Suzanne Somers hosted a small gathering of us at the American Academy of Anti-Aging Medicine (A4M) at our conference in Vegas last December 2013. I got to meet her personally and I found her to be exactly as we see her on television…genuine, down to earth, and totally committed to the alternative medicine and preventive health. In Suzanne's words:

"Forever Health™ provides a network where patients can connetct with physicians who can help them with Bioidentical Hormone Replacement Therapy (BHRT). Thanks to BHRT, I enjoy robust health, balanced hormones, strong bones, and the energy of someone half my age. So naturally, I am proud to be affiliated with Forever Health."

Benefits of optimizing your hormones bio-identically:

- □ Improve mental clarity, focus, and memory
- □ Accelerate fat burning and increase weight loss
- □ Decrease depression and anxiety/ stress
- □ Restore/increase libido
- □ Reduce PMS symptoms, hot flashes, menstrual bleeding, and painful menses
- □ Decrease risk of breast and colon cancer
- □ Improve energy and enhanced mood
- □ Decrease Heart Disease by decreasing LDL and increasing HDL
- □ Prevent or slow osteoporosis and lower the risk of hip fractures
- □ Decrease or delay Alzheimer's or dementia
- □ Improve work productivity
- □ Enhance the immune system

- □ Increase collagen, leading to decreased wrinkles and smoother, more elastic skin

- □ Increase lean body mass (muscles) and improve sleep

....

5. CUSTOMIZED VITAMIN & IV NUTRITION

Customized vitamin therapy is important. Each individual has unique body requirements and different nutritional needs. We can use your medical history, the results of your physical, and your laboratory findings to find out where you are deficient in vitamins, minerals, herbs, amino acids, enzymes, and other nutritional supplements, in order to compound your own personalized nutritional pack. If you tried to make an omelet without eggs, you'd find it impossible. In the same way, your body needs to have all the nutritional supplements, vitamins, enzymes, and minerals to make the hormones, proteins, cofactors, and other vital body processes. We can optimize these nutritional supplements to help you reverse or slow down the aging process and improve other health conditions.

The way in which you receive your nutrients impacts on how effective they will be. Intravenous (IV) nutrition is a method of administering nutrients that is more efficient than ingesting pills, due to limitations of the digestive process. With IV nutrition, the nutrients flow directly into your bloodstream, allowing for a higher rate of absorption. IV nutrition is useful in cases where a patient needs to overcome a virus, whose elimination may require a higher level of a particular vitamin. This level is attainable with IV nutrition, but not with medicine consumed orally. With IV nutrition, vitamins, minerals, amino acids, and other nutrients are slowly administered via a small needle in your vein.

Many illnesses and medical conditions associated with digestive disturbances, such as malabsorption, food sensitivities, and leaky gut syndrome, cause the body to fail at absorbing many crucial nutrients. Stressful situations can cause the body to use certain nutrients at a faster rate or require higher amounts for proper healing. Some common medications deplete the body's supply of particular nutrients, creating deficiencies over time. When nutrients are delivered intravenously, the digestive system is bypassed and 100 percent nutrient absorption is achieved. Introducing nutrients intravenously opens circulation to the cells of your body so that they can easily obtain the nutrients needed to repair, heal, and function.

IV nutritional therapy can be used to treat the following conditions:

- Adrenal fatigue
- Stress
- Fibromyalgia
- Chronic fatigue syndrome
- Depression
- Asthma
- Infection
- Weak immune response
- Immunotoxicity
- Bronchitis
- Decrease recovery time from illness/injury
- Detoxify free radicals and heavy metal
- Cancer

□ Nutritional imbalances in sports or athletes

□ Malnutrition or preop for surgical procedures.

FEELING YOUNGER

We've talked about ways to make you look better and to help your body functions return to their optimal, youthful levels. But there's more to it than that, of course. In order to start feeling younger, we'll have to eliminate stress in order to decrease inflammation in your body. We have to optimize your hormones and neurotransmitters. Your minerals, vitamins, enzymes, and antioxidants have to be optimized. Your environmental allergies and food sensitivities have to be corrected. Finally, your pain has to be eliminated.

At the Wellness and Aesthetics Medical Center, this is paramount to achieving our goal of growing younger. It is the primary reason our patients come to us. Mary, my office manager, commented that we have become a "sex clinic," and in some respects, she is correct: Patients who are not feeling well have no interest in sex. As soon as they begin to feel better, their focus turns to sex. *Healthy* patients have their natural sexual appetites restored.

LOWER STRESS, LOWER INFLAMMATION

What does a positive attitude have to do with decreasing inflammation? Psychiatrists at King's College in London found that people who were physically or sexually abused as children are twice as likely to have significant levels of CRP (C-Reactive Protein, which causes cardiac inflammation and risk of heart attack). This explains why abused children show a higher incident of heart disease and diabetes as adults. The stress of ongoing abuse produces inflammation that will have repercussions later in life.

"Inflammation is a natural response to physical trauma, such as cutting yourself or getting an infection," explains psychiatrist Andrea Danese. "But psychological stress can also trigger inflammation, since stress is really the anticipation of pain."

We all suffer from stress. Unhealthy stress levels can lead to anxiety, hypertension, physical pain, obesity, heart disease, diabetes, physical and mental illnesses, and a whole host of other problems. Stress can be defined as the sum of physical and mental responses to an unacceptable experience. By this definition, stress is a response that includes both physical and mental components.

What causes stress and anxiety? Such things as financial problems, jobs, health concerns, long commutes, heavy traffic, and long working hours are all factors. A recent poll shows that about 75 percent of people in the United States and Canada say they feel stress on a daily basis, and feel their lives are beyond their control. Stress can lead to drug and alcohol abuse.

The fact is that stressors are not going away. Bills will continue to increase. Prices will keep rising. The job market will continue to be depressed. This can and does affect your life, your job, and your children's future. Fortunately, even though you can't change the world around you, you have it within your power to control its impact on your stress levels, and to ensure that it does not interfere with your life or steal your health.

Here are some effective stress management techniques, along with some critical information that will help you combat the stresses in your life:

Identify the stressors in your life

Unknown to many of us, the roots of most of our stress lie within ourselves, in our habits, behaviors, and thought processes. For instance, if you do not learn how to say "No," work will continue to be sent your way. Procrastinating and allowing things to pile up will stress you out. Find ways to take care of stuff now. If you do not control your habit of flying off the handle at the slightest thing, your relationships will continue to be strained. And if you do not break your habit of worrying over the small things or trying to take control of everything and everyone in your life, you will always be stressed out. Take 30 minutes to think about what stresses you out during the day. What weekly occurrences stress you out? What people, activities, or things cause stress in your life? Make a Top 10 list, see which of them can be eliminated, and take action to weed them out.

Evaluate your coping mechanisms

Some stress-busting methods may work in the short run, but actually end up causing severe physical and emotional damage in the long run.

....

Dangerous means of coping with stress

Take a close look at yourself and find out if you are prone to lapsing into any of these:

- Smoking and/or drinking excessively
- Popping pills or taking drugs
- Binge eating or starving yourself
- Shutting out all human contact and/or spending too many mindless hours in front of the television or computer
- Immersing yourself in overwork to escape responsibilities

       ▫ Procrastinating on critical tasks, and/or venting your anger and frustration on others.

Shun these debilitating habits, and instead learn how to cope in a healthy manner.

....

LEARN HOW TO AVOID UNNECESSARY STRESS.

Eight important steps toward taking control of your life.

- **Be prepared to say "No."** Accept that it is perfectly okay to want to avoid certain people—and do so. Find ways around doing non-critical tasks that stress you out, like switching to online shopping if store queues bother you, or if you do not want to deal with finding a parking space or confronting freeway traffic. And finally, sort out your priorities, because some tasks can always be put off until the next day.

- **Eliminate things that drain your energy**. If you've analyzed your life and found things that stress you out, you might have also noticed things that drain your energy. Certain things in our life just cause us to be more exhausted than others, with less value. Identify them, and cut them out. You'll have much more energy and much less stress.

- **Avoid difficult people**. If you take a minute to think about it, you can identify all the people in your life (bosses, coworkers, customers, friends, family, etc.) who make your life more difficult. Cut them out of your life.

- **Try and alter a stressful situation.** Most stressful situations are not beyond your control if only you convey to these other people that are attributable to your stress in regards to how you are feeling. You need to be a little more assertive and demand that you be allowed more time and space. And then work hard to manage your time in the most effective manner. Most of the time, a compromising attitude and not trying to be perfect also help counter stress admirably. We all have many commitments in our life, starting with work but also including commitments related to kids, our spouses, things to do at home, other family, civic, side work, religious, hobbies, online activities, and more. Consider each of them, the amount of stress they provide, and the value you get out of them. Edit brutally, and take steps today to remove the ones that stress you out the most.

- **Take time out to relax**. It's important to take mini-breaks during your workday. Stop what you're doing, massage your shoulders and neck and head and hands and arms, get up and stretch, walk around, drink some water. Go outside and appreciate the fresh air and the beautiful sky. Talk to someone you like. Life doesn't have to be all about productivity. You should also avoid using online activity too much as your de-stressing activity—get away from the computer to relax.

- **Adapt to the stressor.** If the above two ploys—trying to avoid or altering a stressful situation—do not work out, gracefully accept that some things are beyond your control. Adopt a positive attitude, lower your expectations a bit, and re-orient your perspective to find the silver lining in the cloud. Whether you see a glass as half-empty or half-full will ultimately determine how well you adapt to the stressor.

- **Play.** Remember those wise words. All work and no play made Jack a dull boy—which will only contribute to your stress. Take time out to have fun, indulge in activities you love most, and reach out and connect to the people you cherish. There is not any greater stress-buster than play.

- **Follow a healthy lifestyle.** There are tons of scientific studies to prove that regular exercise, a healthy diet, and a solid night's sleep equip your body and mind to cope with stress.

NUTRITION

Nutrition is the provision that cells and organisms need to support life. Many common health problems can be prevented or alleviated with a healthy diet. The diet of an organism is what it eats. Medications, vitamin interaction, soil depletion, need for more antioxidants, stress, age, lifestyle, and genetics all play a role in determining which nutrients are right for you.

And, unfortunately, in our current state, food is not enough to keep us nutritionally well.

Why can't I get the nutrients I need from food?

- The soil is depleted of many minerals such as zinc and magnesium.

- Fruits and vegetables begin to lose their nutritional value immediately after picking. Asparagus stored for one week loses up to 90 percent of its vitamin C.

- The milling of grains removes 26 essential nutrients and much of the fiber.

- The nutrients in your food may not be in the form that is bioavailable.

- Processing (blanching, sterilizing, canning, and freezing) all decrease the nutritional value of the food you eat.

- The longer you cook the fruits and vegetables, the fewer nutrients remain. Therefore, eat most of them raw or lightly steamed.

Additionally, nutrients are affected by free radical production from electronic appliances (television screens, cell phones, computer screens, hair dryers, microwave, airplane trips, florescent lights, etc.). They are also affected by antioxidants if they are not balanced.

How do we eat?

Paradoxically, we residents of one of the richest nations in the world don't eat that well, due mostly to our own bad choices. The Second National Health and Nutrition Examination (NHANES II) survey revealed:

- Fewer than 10% of Americans consume five servings of fruits and vegetables a day
- 40% had no daily fruit or fruit juice
- 50% had no garden vegetable in a day
- 70% had no fruit or vegetable rich in vitamin C in a day
- 80% had no daily fruit or vegetable rich in carotenoids

Foods can affect your medication

Even otherwise-innocuous and healthy foods can create dangerous interactions when consumed by people on certain medications.

Grapefruit, for instance, may increase the risk of side effects of the following medications.

- Calcium-channel blockers if taken with grapefruit can decrease blood pressure, cause flushing, headache, and increased heart rate.

- Grapefruit increases the levels of quinidine.

- Grapefruit can cause irregular heart rhythms if you are taking terfenadine.

- Grapefruit increases estrogen levels for both men and women.

- If you are taking cyclosporine, grapefruit increases the levels and can cause kidney and liver toxicity.

- Grapefruit increases the level of caffeine in your body and can cause nervousness and insomnia.

- If you are taking a sedative (benzodiazepine), grapefruit can increase levels of the medication.

- If you are taking fexofenadine, grapefruit decreases the absorption of the medication.

- If you are taking carbamazepine, grapefruit can increase levels, which may lead to nausea, tremors, drowsiness, dizziness, or agitation.

- Grapefruit delays the absorption of Viagra.

- Grapefruit increases the levels of warfarin.

- If you are taking amiodarone, grapefruit may elevate blood levels and you may have nausea, drowsiness, tremors, or agitation.

- If you are taking statin drugs, grapefruit may increase the medication level.

- Grapefruit and naprosyn taken together may cause hives.

- If you are taking a macrolide antibiotic, grapefruit will decrease its absorption.

Animals know by instinct what to eat and drink. Man has largely lost his powers of instinct. Therefore, man needs nutritional knowledge, and an animal doesn't. Unfortunately, nutrition is barely touched on in medical schools. There is no research money available for the study of nutrition. Seemingly, no one in the medical industry wants to tackle the nutrition problem. Why? One might reasonably deduct that it's because good nutrition keeps us healthy; therefore, we will not need physicians, drug companies, health insurance companies, laboratories, synthetic food industry, and the FDA. The whole $3 trillion health industry would crumble.

Another under-researched and under-treated area of medical science is inflammation—even though there's a substantial body of evidence that it's the root cause of much of what ails us. In the next chapter, we'll talk about inflammation's causes and cures.

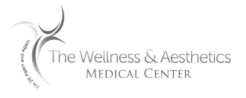
Chapter Three

INFLAMMATION

*I*n order to understand the effects of inflammation on your body, let us first define the term. Inflammation is part of the complex biological response of vascular tissues to harmful stimuli, such as pathogen, damaged cells, or irritants. Inflammation is a protective attempt by the organism to remove the injurious stimuli and to initiate the healing process. Inflammation is the activation of the immune system in response to infection, irritation, or injury. It is characterized by an influx of white blood cells, redness, heat, swelling, pain, and dysfunction of the organs involved. Inflammation has different names when it appears in different parts of the body. Infection is one of multiple causes of inflammation. Without inflammation, wounds and infections would never heal. Similarly, progressive destruction of the tissue would compromise the survival of the organism.

Chronic inflammation can also lead to a host of diseases, such as arthritis, diabetes, heart disease, irritable bowel syndrome, Alzheimer's disease, Parkinson's disease, hypertension, depression, anxiety, chronic pain, asthma, cancer, and many others. It is for that reason that the body closely regulates inflammation.

Most allergy and asthma sufferers are familiar with rhinitis (inflammation of the nose), sinusitis (inflammation of the sinuses), and asthma (inflammation of the airways). Inflammation is also behind arthritis (inflammation of the joints) and dermatitis (inflammation of the skin). In the case of allergies, the immune system responds to the presence of an allergen (a normally harmless substance to which it has become overly sensitive). Allergens bind to antibodies, which trigger the release of chemicals like histamine that result in allergy symptoms. In the case of asthma, inflammation causes the airways to swell, making it difficult to breathe.

As the initial response that fires up the immune system, inflammation is the crucial first step in fighting off infection and healing wounds. When inflammation persists, the immune system is overtaxed. This leads to chronic inflammation and can lead to chronic disease. Foods that increase inflammation are Omega 6 (vegetable oil), refined carbohydrates, trans fats, iron, and alpha-tocopherol.

Inflammation & Alzheimer's disease

In the journal *Neurology* in 1997, neurologists presented research that people who had been regularly taking anti-inflammatory medicine like Ibuprofen had much lower rates of Alzheimer's disease. In the *New England Journal of Medicine* in 2001, a study showed an 80 percent reduction in risk of Alzheimer's among those taking anti-inflammatory medicines daily for two years. Linda Van Eldik, neurobiologist at Northwestern University School of Medicine, explains that whenever the brain is injured or irritated, glial cells pump out cytokines (chemical signals) to begin the inflammatory process. However, "in chronic neurodegenerative diseases like Alzheimer's, these glial cells are active too high or too long or both."

Inflammation & heart disease

Inflammation also plays a role in heart disease, because the immune system attacks LDL, the so-called "bad" cholesterol, which has been embedded in arterial walls. Ongoing inflammation eventually damages the arteries, which can cause them to burst. Inflammation is so closely associated with heart disease that a CRP (C-reactive protein) is used to assess a person's risk of heart attack. Research shows that CRP can predict the risk of heart attack and stroke as well or better than can cholesterol levels.

Inflammation & diabetes

Inflammation has been linked to diabetes, as well. In Type 1 diabetes, the immune system attacks the cells that make insulin. Children who have allergies are less likely to develop Type 1 diabetes. "Children with Type 1 diabetes are less likely to get asthma, eczema, or hay fever," says pediatrician Dr. Alan Greene, MD. "And the reverse is true, that those with asthma, eczema, or hay fever are less likely to get Type 1 diabetes."

Type II diabetes is also linked to inflammation, as chronic inflammation releases TNF (tumor necrosis factor), which makes cells more resistant to insulin.

Inflammation & cancer

"Although there is plenty of evidence that chronic inflammation can promote cancer, the cause of this relationship is not understood," says Alexander Hoffmann, an assistant professor of chemistry and biochemistry at U.C. San Diego, who led the study. "We have identified a basic cellular mechanism that we think may be linking chronic inflammation and cancer."

A protein called p100 allows communication between the inflammation and development processes. Some amount of dialogue is beneficial, but too much dialogue (which results from chronic inflammation) can lead to unrestrained development (cancer). According to Hoffman, "studies with animals have shown that a little inflammation is necessary for the normal development of the immune system and other organ systems. We discovered that the protein p100 provides the cell with a way in which inflammation can influence development. In the case of chronic inflammation, the presence of too much p100 may over activate the developmental pathway, resulting in cancer."

How to decrease chronic inflammation

Aspirin is one of the oldest anti-inflammatory medications. Many people take it to prevent heart attack and stroke. Ibuprofen may help protect against Alzheimer's disease, but NSAIDs (non-steroidal anti-inflammatory agents), such as aspirin and ibuprofen, can have significant side effects, such as liver damage. You can also lower inflammation levels through lifestyle changes. The best way is through nutrition, exercise, sleep, and a positive attitude.

CHRONIC FATIGUE SYNDROME & FIBROMYALGIA

Melissa is a 42-year-old female and the mother of three teenagers. Her husband was a prominent businessman in Laredo, Texas. She was healthy until the birth of her third child 13 years ago. After the birth of the child, she was diagnosed with postpartum depression. She started suffering from insomnia and being tired during the day. She started having muscle and joint pains as well as headaches. She went to several doctors, but received no help from them. She became so fatigued that she could not return to her job. Her relationship with her spouse deteriorated. After six years of trying to get help, she was on multiple medications. She had gained 60 pounds. She was cold all the time.

Finally, four years ago, her husband divorced her. She felt hopeless. She started to give up on life. At one point, she contemplated suicide. She continued to take all her medication. She had severe pain every day. Two years ago, a friend who was a patient at the Wellness and Aesthetics Medical Center in San Antonio, Texas, recommended it to her.

On a rainy day in November 2011, I evaluated Melissa. After a battery of tests in my office, Melissa and I talked for 90 minutes. I answered all of her questions, and explained to her our goal of optimization, finding the cause of her problems and eradicating them. We discussed how our bodies function, and some of the medical myths I talked about in an earlier chapter. She kept looking at her watch. Finally, I asked if she needed to leave. She said no doctor has ever spent so much time with her and explained so much to her. I explained that I only schedule four patients per day and that the morning was reserved for her, since she was a new patient. She was very pleased. We devised a six-month plan to fix her problem.

Two weeks later, she called and told me that she felt much better. She said her pain had diminished. In two months, she had lost 20 pounds, and her sleep had improved. Her energy was significantly improved, and her sex drive was up. She had even started a new job.

Chronic Fatigue Syndrome (CFS) is a chronic disorder characterized by widespread musculoskeletal pain, fatigue, and multiple tender points that occur in precise, localized areas, particularly in the neck, spine, shoulders, and hips. It may cause sleep disturbances, morning stiffness, irritable bowel syndrome, anxiety and other symptoms. For many decades, fibromyalgia syndrome was considered an emotional problem, created by anxious or depressed persons. This theory was debunked in the 1970s, mainly due to the fact that most fibromyalgia patients do not have emotional problems (as the root cause of the condition, that is; many ultimately do as a result of chronic pain).

Fibromyalgia Syndrome (FMS) may resemble a post-viral state. This similarity is the reason experts of FMS and CFS believe these two syndromes may be the same. According to the National Fibromyalgia Association, there are 15–20 million people who suffer from fibromyalgia. Ninety percent are women. The problem usually begins between 20–30 years of age. The CDC estimates there are more than 5 million with fibromyalgia and 1–4 million with chronic fatigue syndrome and immune dysfunction syndrome (CFIDS). These patients suffer from debilitating fatigue, joint pain, muscle weakness, headaches, insomnia, mental fog, and depression. Seventy percent of the patients consider themselves to be disabled. Most, if not all, report sleep disturbances.

There are no diagnostic tests or real treatment for these medical diagnoses. They are considered diagnoses of exclusion. Patients have to endure the symptoms and are placed on multiple drugs to treat the symptoms (band-aids).

Fibromyalgia derives from the Latin words *fibro* (fibrous tissue) *myo* (muscle) *algia* (pain). Chronic Fatigue Syndrome comes from overwhelming persistent fatigue. The underlying cause of Fibromyalgia and chronic fatigue syndrome are different but related conditions that share a common symptom—overwhelming fatigue that significantly decreases the quality of your life. The causes of CFS and FMS are still unknown.

CERTAIN TRIGGERS PRECIPITATE THE ONSET. THESE TRIGGERS ARE:

- Viral or bacterial infection.
- A severe injury, or the development of another disorder (rheumatoid arthritis, lupus, or hypothyroidism). They

don't directly cause Fibromyalgia Syndrome, but they may awaken an underlying physiological abnormality that is already present.

- Some evidence also points to a problem with the immune system. Certain immunologic abnormalities are common among people with FMS.

Many women acquire the symptoms at times of hormonal fluxes, as in childbirth, and perimenopausal times. This just happens to correlate with the onset of hypothyroidism in many women. Some evidence also points to a problem with the immune system. Certain immunologic abnormalities are common among people with FMS.

THE SYMPTOMS OF CFS AND FMS ARE CHARACTERIZED BY:

- Musculoskeletal pain
- Severe fatigue
- Multiple tender points occurring in localized areas, such as the neck, spine, shoulders, and hips
- Sleep disturbances
- Morning stiffness
- Irritable bowel syndrome/constipation
- Anxiety
- Difficulty concentrating or confusion
- Increased irritability
- Mental fog/fibro fog
- Bloating
- Painful menses

- Depression and anxiety
- Panic attacks, nausea, dizziness, and sore throat
- Shortness of breath, memory loss, chest pain
- Increased allergy symptoms
- Blurred vision, light sensitivities, weight loss or gain
- Numbness or tingling in extremities, cold extremities, chronic cough
- Chills and night sweats

Ways of managing CFS and FMS

Treatments for Fibromyalgia Syndrome and Chronic Fatigue Syndrome are aimed at improving the quality of sleep and in reducing pain commonly experienced by sufferers. Medications that boost the body's level of serotonin and norepinephrine are commonly prescribed.

Commonly used treatments:

- Acupressure
- Acupuncture
- Physical Therapy
- Relaxation/biofeedback techniques
- Chiropractic care
- Therapeutic massage
- Ayurvedic medicine
- Herbal teas, supplements, etc.
- Naturopathic medicine
- Osteopathy

- ▫ Physiotherapy

- ▫ Homeopathy

The list of treatments does not stop there. The treatments of FMS and CFS differ, just like the causes. Other management strategies include:

- Consuming 50 percent of diet from raw food (e.g., fruits, vegetables, whole grains, raw nuts and seeds)

- Taking probiotics that contain acidophilus

- Increasing water consumption

- Increasing fiber to keep bowels moving

- Avoiding highly processed foods that deplete the body of magnesium, which leads to fatigue

- Getting adequate sleep and rest

- Maintaining a moderate exercise program

In 2007, the FDA approved Lyrica for the treatment of FMS. Pfizer originally made it for the treatment of seizure. The FDA for treatment of fibromyalgia then approved Cymbalta, made by Eli Lilly and Company. These drugs are minimally effective in reducing fibromyalgia pain. Their side effects include nausea, weight gain, constipation, dizziness, blurred vision, and decreased concentration, drowsiness, swelling of hands and feet, and suicidal plans. Some of these side effects are symptoms of fibromyalgia.

The pain of fibromyalgia and the fatigue associated with chronic fatigue syndrome are often misinterpreted as being caused by another disorder. In point of fact, the symptoms are identical to those of hypothyroidism. Treatment with desiccated thyroid (amour thyroid) has been effective. The main symptom of fibromyalgia is widespread pain. The main symptom of chronic fatigue syndrome is debilitating fatigue.

At the Wellness and Aesthetics Medical Center, we treat the hypothyroidism, clean up the gut (with a gluten-free, yeast-free diet), give large doses of probiotics, and support the adrenals. Miraculously, our patients get better.

OBESITY AND INFLAMMATION

Martha is a 46-year-old mother of two teenage sons living in Eagle Pass, Texas. All four members of the family were markedly obese. She heard about the Wellness and Aesthetics Medical Center from another weight-loss patient. Martha and her family visited us in San Antonio.

After a full evaluation with in-clinic testing and a 60-minute discussion with me, I placed the entire family on a weight reduction program. They were so inspired that on their return home, they emptied their kitchen of all the processed and poor-nutrition food. Over the next six months, they lost a combined 300 pounds. Both teenagers now weigh less than 160 pounds. Mom has gone from 210 lbs to 130, and Dad is down to 180 lbs from 260.

Martha's situation is hardly unique. Obesity is a burgeoning epidemic, fueled by our addiction to "fast" foods, processed foods, and unhealthy diets. The average U.S. caloric consumption has gone from 1,980 calories in 1960 to 3,766 in 2009. More than 200 million Americans are overweight or obese. Moreover, 68 percent are overweight and 34 percent obese. Twenty percent of children were obese in 2010. In the past 20 years, diabetes has increased 10-fold, clearly as a result of the obesity epidemic.

What relationship does obesity have to inflammation? In 2006, Tufts University scientist Andrew Greenberg found that as fat cells reach their maximum size, they break down and die. Specialized immune cells called macrophages rush in to clean up the debris. Macrophages are responsible for most of the inflammatory chemicals released in fat tissue. "When fat cells die, macrophages surround the dead lipids the same way white cells surround a wooden splinter in your skin," Greenberg wrote. "The immune system is essentially surrounding and sequestering the dead fat cells and gorging on the leftover lipids and cellular debris." Inflammation from excess fat cells explains why obesity complicates arthritis, insulin resistance, diabetes, and heart disease. Exercising regularly can decrease the inflammation.

Though obesity is considered a medical problem causing inflammation and a major catalysis for diabetes, hypertension, heart disease, depression, cancer, CVA, arthritis, Alzheimer's disease, Chronic Fatigue Syndrome, and infertility, most physicians surveyed expressed low confidence in their ability to treat it. Most reported low or no exposure to systematic training in the treatment of obesity. Physicians indicated that they rarely formally refer their obese patients to weight-loss programs. They report lack of time in busy practices and lack of resources and tools available.

The largest endocrine organ in our body is now fat. It can support or dampen the immune system, and can cause blood vessels to constrict, leading to increased blood pressure (hypertension). Fat controls how energy is stored and how and when it is mobilized. It stores increasing amount of toxins, which increases inflammation.

Hormones, which are made and regulated by fat, include:

- Adiponectin—Modulates glucose regulation and fatty acid catabolism.

- Resistin—Involved in insulin resistance. Serum Resistin levels increase with increased obesity.

- Plasminogen Activator Inhibitor (PAL-1)—Linked to increased occurrence of thrombosis. Inflammatory conditions plays significant role in progression to fibrosis.

- TNF-α (Tumor Necrosis Factor – α)—Primary role is to regulate immune cells and dysregulation leads to: Alzheimer's, cancer, major depression, and irritable bowel syndrome (IBS).

- IL-6 (Interluken-6)—Acts as a pro-inflammatory and anti-inflammatory cytokine. Extremely important in fever and acute phase response.

- Estradiol—Aids in development of secondary sex characteristics, body shape, bones, joints, and fat deposition. In men, increased levels lead to decreased sperm count.

- Adipose—The greatest peripheral source of aromatase in both males and females. It increases production of estradiol by converting testosterone in estradiol.

- Leptin—Acts on the hypothalamus to help control appetite. Plays key role in regulating energy intake and expenditure, including appetite and metabolism. The levels of circulating leptin directly reflect the amount of energy stored in the adipose tissue, and are proportional to the body adipose mass. Obese individuals typically produce higher levels of leptin than leaner individuals, yet obese subjects are

resistant to the inhibitory activity that this molecule has on
food intake and on the control of satiety.

....

Evidence and experience point to the fact that there exists a strong correlation between maintaining a healthy weight and controlling inflammation, and that weight and hormone production also are strongly interrelated. Hormonal balance, or symphony, is another little-understood but crucial piece in the overall wellness pictures. In the next chapter, we'll talk about what hormones are, what they do, and how proper balance can help you gain and keep your youth, particularly **Testosterone, Estrogen,** and **Progesterone.**

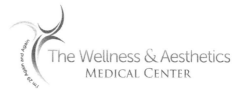
Chapter Four

HORMONES IN HARMONY

arilyn is a 54-year-old female from Dallas, Texas. She is married to a very successful trial lawyer. She has a stressful job, which keeps her on the road three or four days per week. Over the past five years, she had noticed increasing loss of libido, energy, and memory. She has been married to her second husband for 10 years and had noted diminishing sexual desire. To complicate matters, she began having insomnia and decreased work productivity, and had a 30-pound weight gain.

She had visited several doctors who told her that all of this was normal for her age. They checked her blood and told her that her numbers were within normal range. I met Marilyn at Urban Retreat day spa when I was doing a seminar on laser therapy. Marilyn took my card. She later went to my website: www.twaamc.com. She scheduled a visit to The Wellness and Aesthetics Medical Center.

Marilyn had a typical three-hour evaluation at our office (60-90 min with me and 60-90 min in testing and teaching). She was placed on a treatment program, which included testosterone and estrogen pellets, as well as desiccated thyroid and progesterone. She was also placed on nutritional supplements and a gut repair kit. Two weeks later, Marilyn called and reported significant improvement in her symptoms. She comes every three to four months to get her pellets. She claims she has never felt better.

How could hormones make such a difference in a person's wellness? Let's examine the three key hormones, and what they do in our bodies.

TESTOSTERONE

Testosterone is a hormone secreted by the ovaries, adrenal glands, and testes. Both men and woman need it. Women need a much smaller amount and it can sustain a woman's libido and enhance the functions of estrogen. In both males and females, it strengthens bones to help prevent bone loss.

Testosterone is the primary male sex hormone, responsible for male sexual development, and critical in maintaining erectile function, libido, energy levels, mood, and a wide range of other physical functions throughout the body. As with most other hormones, testosterone declines with age. Testosterone levels begin declining when a man is in his early 30s. Although the total testosterone does not drop dramatically, the free testosterone, which is the biologically active testosterone, declines dramatically with age. Because the drop in testosterone is gradual, andropause (male menopause) symptoms appear over a longer period of time as compared to female menopause. Symptoms appear as a gradual decrease in energy; decrease in bone density and muscles; increased visceral fat; depression; decrease in memory and mental focus; and impaired sexual function. Testosterone deficiency has also been linked to hypertension, obesity, and increased heart discase risks.

Benefits of Testosterone Replacement:

- Improves energy and enhances mood
- Enhances libido
- Improves sleep and decreases stress
- Improves cognitive functioning, memory/ mental focus
- Improves work productivity
- Decreases abdominal fat and increases lean body mass
- Improves recovery from exercise
- Improves blood glucose levels
- Balances healthy blood pressure
- Decreases heart disease risk through decreased LDL and increased HDL
- Decreases osteoporosis, lowers risk of hip fracture
- Enhances skin and hair texture
- Decreases or delays Alzheimer's or dementia

Let's talk more specifically about how the presence or absence of testosterone can impact the functions of specific organs in your body. The organ most affected by testosterone is the heart. It is the largest muscle in our body. When you are 20, your heart is like an 18-wheeler pulling a Volkswagen. At 60, your heart is like a Volkswagen pulling an 18-wheeler. Your heart is a muscle that testosterone makes strong at 20. Your heart beats effortlessly, pumping blood. At 60, your testosterone is low, so your heart muscle is weak and atrophied. Therefore, your heart has to work very hard to push blood throughout the body. The increase workload on the heart increases your risk of heart disease. Testosterone protects you from heart disease.

The second organ most affected by testosterone is your brain. Testosterone improves your memory and cognitive function. It decreases your stress level and improves your sleep. Testosterone decreases your risk of getting Alzheimer's disease and dementia. Testosterone improves your work performance by making you more proficient, happier, pleasant to be around, and more energized. Testosterone gives you back that feeling of invincibility that you had when you were 20. Testosterone decreases your belly fat, increases your muscle mass, and increases your bone density (when you are 20 and you fall, you jump up; when you fall and you are 60, you break your hip), and increases your energy level. As a side effect, your libido and sex drive are increased.

Testosterone isn't just for men. In fact, women need it just as much. Testosterone should be optimized in everyone. The benefits are undisputed.

ESTROGEN

There are three types of estrogen found in a female's body: estrone, estradiol, and estriol. The levels of all of these hormones fall dramatically at the onset of menopause. Estrogen is produced in women's ovaries and adrenal glands. An extremely small amount of estrogen is produced in men through the conversion of testosterone.

With the onset of menopause, there is a rapid decline in estrogen, leading to multiple problems (cardiovascular disease, stroke, osteoporosis, dementia, and alzheimer's). Symptoms characteristic of female menopause are hot flashes, insomnia, vaginal dryness, bladder problems, difficulty concentrating, and anxiety. Estrogen lowers total blood cholesterol and raises HDL (good cholesterol). While estrogen protects the heart, it also protects the brain from cognitive impairments.

Estrogen can protect a woman against many of the diseases of aging, and post-menopausal women on estrogen typically feel better and stay healthier. Unfortunately, most of the estrogen that is prescribed to women is synthetic estrogen, an estrogen that is not natural to the human body. Because of this, many women develop side effects. It is best to avoid synthetic estrogens and use natural estrogens. Why? Human receptor sites were designed to accept natural estrogen, not the synthetics. Studies have shown that long-term use of synthetic estrogens increases the formation of breast cancer, heart disease, and colon cancer. In contrast, natural estrogen, especially when taken in conjunction with natural progesterone, can protect against breast cancer, heart disease, and colon cancer similar to the way it protects against uterine cancer. The use of estriol, which is a weak estrogen, has been shown to lower the incidence of breast cancer.

Benefits of Estrogen Replacement:

- Decreases risk of breast cancer and colon cancer
- Decreases symptoms of menopause
- Improves vaginal dryness and eliminates bladder problems
- Improves energy and enhances mood
- Enhances libido
- Improves sleep and decreases stress
- Improves cognitive functioning, memory/mental focus
- Improves work productivity
- Decreases abdominal fat and increases lean body mass
- Improved recovery from exercise

- Improved blood glucose levels
- Balances healthy blood pressure
- Decreases heart disease by decreasing LDL and increasing HDL
- Decreases osteoporosis, and lowers risk of hip fracture
- Increases collagen leading to decreased wrinkles and smoother, better skin
- Decrease or delays onset of Alzheimer's and dementia

Natural (bioidentical) estrogen and progesterone are a woman's youth. If she desires to remain young and vibrant, she needs to optimize them. Estrogen and progesterone work together in a symphony to maintain a woman's youth, health, energy, sexual appeal, and aesthetics. Together, they protect her from breast cancer, colon cancer, and heart disease, keep her wrinkle free, maintain her vaginal lubrication, her bone density, protect her memory and cognitive functions and her hair and nails. They enhance her libido, energy, mood, and decrease premenstrual symptoms. Estrogen and progesterone optimization is a must for EVERY woman.

PROGESTERONE

Progesterone is a hormone produced by the ovaries and adrenal glands and functions to balance the effects of estrogen. Natural progesterone enhances the action of estrogen, as these hormones work together to maintain a normal hormone balance. The ovaries begin producing progesterone around puberty. Progesterone and estrogen maintain a harmonious relationship through menopause. Progesterone levels increase sharply after ovulation at about day 14. Levels drop four days prior to menstruation if the egg is not fertilized. Progesterone's primary role during this period is to help make the uterus ready for implantation of a new embryo and protection of the fetus throughout the nine months of human gestation. If the egg is not fertilized, progesterone production temporarily ceases, and the uterus sheds its endometrial lining.

Suboptimal levels of progesterone causes disease processes similar to estrogen, which include depression, anxiety, irritability, mood swings, insomnia, osteoporosis, heart disease, decrease in libido, and a significantly diminished quality of life. The combination of natural progesterone and estrogen can keep a woman healthy and energized.

....

Benefits of Progesterone Replacement:

- Precursor to the sex hormones (estrogen and testosterone)
- Maintains uterus lining
- Promotes the survival of the embryo and fetus throughout gestation
- Protects against fibrocystic breasts
- Natural diuretic, lowers cholesterol
- Balances mood, enhance sleep
- Aids thyroid hormone action
- Supports healthy blood clotting
- Helps healthy blood sugar levels
- Protects against breast cancer
- Sustains strong bones
- Helps balance estrogen
- Lowers blood pressure

....

DHEA

Dehydroepiandrosterone DHEA is the most abundant hormone in our body. It is made by the adrenal gland and is converted into testosterone and estradiol. Like most other hormones, it peaks between ages 25 and 35, and then declines rapidly. The amount of DHEA in your system at 50 is a fraction of its peak level. It helps with sexual desire, bone density, mood, skin texture, and healthy body weight. DHEA is considered the "anti-aging hormone" because of it profound effect on skin optimization, conversion to testosterone and estradiol, and stimulation of IGF-1. It is relatively inexpensive and can be purchased with or without a prescription.

Benefits of DHEA Replacement:

- Improves energy and enhances mood
- Enhances libido
- Improves sleep and decreases stress
- Improves cognitive functioning, memory/mental focus
- Improves work productivity
- Decreases abdominal fat and increases lean body mass
- Improves recovery from exercise
- Improves blood glucose levels and insulin resistance
- Improvement in depression
- Decreases heart disease by decreasing LDL and increasing HDL
- Decreases osteoporosis, improves bone density, and lowers risk of hip fracture
- Enhances skin and hair texture, improves collagen

- □ Improves wound healing
- □ Protects from cancer
- □ Produces IGF-1 (growth hormone)
- □ Suppresses interleukin-6, which suppresses chronic inflammatory disorders

OXYTOCIN

Oxytocin (the "cuddle" or "bonding" hormone) is produced by the posterior pituitary. It is a peptide of nine amino acids. It acts as a neuromodulator in the brain and promotes a feeling of happiness, love, and sexual bonding. It improves sexual arousal and orgasm. Oxytocin curbs your appetite and promotes a sense of well-being.

Benefits of Oxytocin Replacement:

- □ Improves energy and enhances mood
- □ Enhances libido
- □ Improves sleep and decreases stress
- □ Helps with lactation during breastfeeding
- □ Important for cervical dilation before birth
- □ Improves social bonding and wound healing
- □ Improves sexual arousal and orgasm
- □ May help in autism
- □ Improves trust and reduces fear
- □ Promotes romantic attraction
- □ Affects generosity by increasing empathy

        ▫ Facilitates learning and memory, specifically for social information

PREGNENOLONE

Pregnenolone (the "mother hormone" or "memory hormone") is synthesized from cholesterol and made by the adrenals. It makes a multitude of other hormones (including DHEA, progesterone, estrogen, testosterone, and cortisol). It promotes sexual arousal and improves orgasm. It improves memory 100 times more than DHEA. Low levels of pregnenolone can lead to multiple hormonal deficiency.

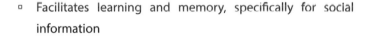

Benefits of Pregnenolone Replacement:

        ▫ Improves energy and enhances mood

        ▫ Enhances libido and orgasm

        ▫ Improves sleep and decreases stress

        ▫ Improves memory, concentration, and cognitive function

        ▫ Decreases depression and stress

        ▫ Improves immune, cardiac, neurological, dermatological, and sexual function

THYROID, GROWTH HORMONE, AND CORTISOL

Thyroid hormone is a metabolic hormone secreted by the thyroid gland. There are three types of thyroid hormones, Thyroxine (T4), Triiodothyronine (T3), and T2. T4 is inactive. T3 is the active hormone. T2 increases metabolic rate of your muscles and fat tissue. Thyroid hormones control the growth, differentiation, and metabolism of each cell in the body. They also control how fast our body uses the fuel that we consume, particularly carbohydrates and fat. This helps to regulate our body temperature and fat percentage. About 93 percent of thyroid hormone production is T4, the inactive thyroid hormone that is typically held in reserve by the body. T3 makes up only 7 percent of the thyroid hormone and is the active hormone that the body uses to function. T4 is converted into T3 by the liver, kidney, and our cells when thyroid hormone is needed. Our good bacterial flora of the gut converts 20 percent of T4 to T3. Testosterone and progesterone converts T4 to T3 also.

The release of the thyroid hormones is controlled by the thyroid-stimulating hormone (TSH), which is produced in the pituitary gland. Low-circulating levels of thyroid hormone are detected by the hypothalamus, which then instructs the pituitary to release TSH. When sufficient amounts of thyroid hormone are circulating, the hypothalamus communicates with the pituitary to stop or slow down. Because of this complicated feedback loop, high levels of TSH in the blood often means the pituitary is trying to stimulate thyroid hormone production, but the thyroid gland is not responding. This condition is known as hypothyroidism.

Thyroid Hormone Benefits:

- Regulates temperature, metabolism and cerebral function
- Increases energy, body temperature, and warmth
- Increases fat breakdown resulting in decreased weight and lower cholesterol
- Protects against cardiovascular ailments
- Improves cerebral metabolism
- Supports cognitive function

□ Relieves symptoms of thin sparse hair, dry skin, and thin
nails

What does all this mean in terms of how you function and feel?
Thyroid Hormone (T3) is your spark plug. You will not burn fat if
your T3 is low. It doesn't matter how much you eat, you will have no
energy, feel cold, and gain weight if your T3 level is low.

What is hypothyroidism?

- Inadequate production of hormone by the thyroid gland.

- Inadequate absorption of thyroid hormone by our cells.

Your thyroid gland works in concert with your hypothalamus and
your pituitary gland to control your body's energy needs. In response
to stressors and changes in temperature, your hypothalamus produces
thyrotropin-releasing hormone (TRH), which tells the pituitary
gland to respond. The pituitary gland releases TSH (thyroid stimulating hormone), which tells the thyroid gland to secrete thyroid
hormone. If your thyroid hormones were low, your cells would not
be able to burn fat for energy. You can take a car to the gas station
and filled it up with gas but the car will not drive until you ignite the
engine.

Low thyroid levels lead to increased fatigue, increased weight
gain, increased depression, problems sleeping, brain fog, and lots of
other issues. Your cells need energy to do their work. The brain uses
up 20 percent of the energy that the body produces. Therefore, when
your thyroid hormone is low, your brain is significantly affected more
than your other organs, leading to problems with concentration,
memory, cognitive function, and brain fog.

The cost of health care has increased tenfold since 1980. In 1980, the cost of health care was $256 billion; today it is more than $2.6 trillion. In America, 67 percent of the population is overweight and 33 percent is obese. In France, the obesity rate is 8 percent, and in Italy, 9 percent. Low thyroid hormone levels lead to obesity, which in turn leads to Type 2 diabetes. That leads to hypertension, which leads to coronary artery disease, degenerative joint disease, Alzheimer's disease, and cancer.

When you go to the doctor and say, "Doc, I feel cold, tired, and rundown; I have no energy, I'm gaining weight, and my hair is falling out," he or she is likely as not to tell you that you're simply depressed. He does not check your thyroid function, or checks it and says you are in the normal range, so it cannot be your thyroid. The test (your TSH) is rigged so that 95 percent of the tests come back as normal, and only 5 percent abnormal. As we have told you already, 67 percent of Americans are overweight and 33 percent are obese; therefore, 95 percent of Americans cannot have normal thyroid functions. It is easier to write a prescription for synthetic medication than to think about the cause, which would cost more time and effort on the physician's part.

The sad fact, as I've observed, is that doctors by and large merely put band-aids on patients; they do not try to find the underlying cause of the problem and fix it. Insurance companies control the doctor (our patients and our income). Insurance companies and the pharmaceutical industry control the medical societies, with the academic medical professors receive payments from big pharma and insurance companies. Insurance companies and big pharma have no interest in promoting natural approaches to health. A healthy public requires less health care. The insurance company and big pharma would much rather have an unhealthy public so that they can charge more in premium payments and have you buy more synthetic drugs. As cynical as that may sound, you need only look around you to see the evidence that this is so.

....

Symptoms of Hypothyroidism:

- Fatigue
- Weight gain
- Cold hands and feet
- Low body temperature
- Tingling and numbness in extremities
- Problems with mental focus
- Decline in mental sharpness; brain fog
- Brittle fingernails with ridging
- Enlarged thyroid gland
- Insomnia
- Mood swings
- Depressed moods
- Joint and muscle aches and pains
- Irritable bowel syndrome
- Sluggish bowel functions and constipation
- Headaches
- Frequent infections
- Irregular menstrual cycles
- Infertility
- Miscarriages
- Loss of libido

- Hair loss in females

- Loss of the lateral third of the eyebrows

- Enlarged tongue with indentations/ridges

- Elevated cholesterol

- Dry brittle skin

- Low blood pressure

- Decrease sweating

- Hoarseness

- Pale or pasty complexion

- Slow in speech

- Prone to rambling

- Fluid retention

- Allergies

Diagnosing hypothyroidism

Hypothyroidism is defined as inadequate production of thyroid hormone by the thyroid gland or inadequate absorption of thyroid hormones by our cells. The thyroid gland produces two main types of thyroid hormones: T4, which is inactive; and T3, which is active thyroid. Ninety-three percent of the thyroid secreted is T4 and 7 percent is T3. T4 has to be converted in the cells to T3 to be active. Unfortunately, we do not have a test to test how much is converted to T3 in the cell. Testing TSH (thyroid stimulating hormone) is inadequate, because it only reflects the signal to the thyroid to make thyroid hormone; it does not reflect how much thyroid hormone is actually being made.

An accurate diagnosis of hypothyroidism is best made by a good history from the patient, combined with the symptoms and judicious use of testing. Testing for micronutrient deficiencies such as Fe, Zn, Iodine, and Selenium can be helpful. It's important too to check for leaky gut and autoimmune diseases, such as thyroid peroxidase antibodies (TPO) and antithyroglobulin antibodies (ATA)).

What Are the Causes of Hypothyroidism?

- Autoimmune thyroid disease
- Sex hormone imbalance and decline
- Estrogen dominance in women
- Hysterectomy, followed by treatment with only extra synthetic estrogen hormones
- Sex hormone decline in men
- Adrenal fatigue
- Aging and hormonal decline in both females and males
- Fluoride poisoning of the thyroid
- Iron, zinc, selenium, and magnesium deficiency
- Cellular resistance to thyroid hormone
- Surgical removal or radioactive destruction of the thyroid gland
- Synthetic drugs such as beta blockers HTN, and lithium for bipolar disorder

Treatment of hypothyroidism

Hypothyroidism has been treated for over a hundred years with desiccated (dried) thyroid extract (Armour thyroid). This is a combination of T3 and T4 that is the same as that made by the thyroid. But it's the underlining cause of the problem that has to be addressed and repaired, by treating the patient's adrenal fatigue (if that is the problem), treating yeast overgrowth, and repairing leaky gut if auto-immune disease is the problem. It's important too that the patient eat a balanced diet with adequate doses of vitamins and mineral supplementation, and that environmental allergies and food allergies and sensitivities are repaired.

GROWTH HORMONE (GH OR HGH)

Growth hormone (GH or HGH, also known as **somatotropin** or **somatropin**) is a peptide that stimulates growth, cell reproduction, and regeneration in humans and other animals. Growth hormone is a 191-amino acid single-chain polypeptide that is synthesized, stored, and secreted by somatotropic cells within the lateral wings of the anterior pituitary gland. Growth hormone (GH) directs the repair of damaged tissue and cell growth. If your GH had been low when you were 12, you would be several inches shorter than you are. If your GH level is low and you have an injury, GH would direct your body to fix it next week. If your level were optimal, it would direct your body to fix it now. GH optimization is important for your immune system, your energy and mood, your vision, memory, cognitive function, maintenance of your vital organs, and wound healing.

Benefits of Human Growth Hormone Replacement:

- Faster wound healing and stronger bones
- Improves sexual performance
- Healthy maintenance of vital organs
- Lowers risk of heart disease

- Lowers cholesterol and blood pressure
- Reduces body fat and increases muscle mass
- Enhances mood and increases energy level
- Sharpens vision and memory
- Enhances cognitive functioning
- Re-grows your hair, provides smoother and firmer skin
- Enhances immune functioning

CORTISOL

Cortisol is a steroid hormone (glucorticoid) produced by the zona fasciculata of the adrenal cortex. It is released in response to stress and a low level of blood glucorticoid. Its primary functions are to increase blood sugar through gluconeogenesis; suppress the immune system; and aid in fat, protein, and carbohydrate metabolism. It also decreases bone formation. It is the only hormone in your body that increases with age. Low levels can lead to profound fatigue and death. Cortisol is needed to cope with stressors.

Benefits of Cortisol Regulation:

- Balances blood sugar
- Weight control
- Improves immune system response
- Bone turnover rate and protein synthesis
- Stress reaction and sleep
- Mood and thoughts
- Influences testosterone/estrogen ratio

□ Influences DHEA/Insulin ratio

□ Affects pituitary/Thyroid/adrenal system

....

Cortisol is your stress hormone. It helps us cope with stressors and react to life threatening emergencies. If your cortisol levels are low, the smallest stressor can put you over the edge.

INSULIN

Insulin (fat storage hormone) is a peptide hormone produced by beta cells of the pancreas. It is a major hormone, which will lead to death if it is too high or low. Insulin causes cells in the liver, skeletal muscles, and fat to absorb glucose from the blood. In the liver and skeletal muscles, glucose is stored as glycogen, and in fat cells it is stored as triglycerides. Insulin determines if glucose will be burned for energy or stored as fat.

Elevated insulin can lead to hypoglycemia and coma. It will also lead to insulin resistance (Type 2 diabetes) and glucose to be stored as fat. Elevated cortisol increases insulin levels, insulin resistance, and fat storage.

As we've seen, balance is everything when it comes to your health. Having out-of-balance hormones creates a variety of symptoms from minor to serious, and can negatively impact your health and well-being. Hormones working together in perfect balance—hormonal symphony are a key piece in the retrieval and maintenance of your youth.

Next, let's look at the key nutrients that support your body and maintain your youth.

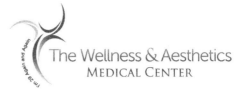
The Wellness & Aesthetics
MEDICAL CENTER

Chapter Five

VITAMINS, MINERALS, AND ANTIOXIDANTS

A s with hormones, your body requires a balance of good, available nutrients to function at its best. Some of them are probably already familiar to you, others you may not have even heard of. Let's dig into these, and discover what each of them does for us—and why we can't do without them.

A **vitamin** is an organic compound required by an organism as a vital nutrient. They occur naturally in both animals and plants. It cannot be synthesized in sufficient quantities by an organism, and must be obtained from the diet. Vitamins are classified by their biological and chemical activity, not their structure.

Vitamins have diverse biochemical functions. Some have hormone-like functions as regulators of mineral metabolism (such as vitamin D), or regulators of cell and tissue growth and differentiation (such as some forms of vitamin A). Vitamins are divided into two categories (fat soluble and water soluble). Fat-soluble vitamins are stored in fat cells (vitamin A, D, E, and K). Water-soluble vitamins (vitamin B and C) are eliminated from the body the same day they are consumed.

The type of vitamins we consume makes a difference. Organic (from a living source—plant or animal) vitamins and minerals are readily absorbed. Inorganic (from a non living source) is very poorly absorbed. Most synthetic vitamins and minerals are from inorganic sources and, therefore, poorly absorbed.

VITAMIN D

Vitamin D is a group of fat-soluble secosteroids responsible for enhancing intestinal absorption of calcium and phosphate. In humans, the most important compounds in this group are vitamin D3 (Cholecalciferol) and vitamin D2 (Ergocalciferol). Cholecalciferol and ergocalciferol can be ingested from the diet and from supplements. The body can also synthesize vitamin D (specifically cholecalciferol) in the skin, from cholesterol, when sun exposure is adequate (hence its nickname, the "sunshine vitamin").

Benefits of Vitamin D Replacement:

- Reduces blood pressure, and CHF
- Reduces risk of infection
- Increases insulin sensitivities
- Reduces circulating cytokines
- Strengthens bone, decreases depression
- Reduces dementia, Alzheimer's, and strokes
- Regulates plasma calcium level
- Reduces risk of autoimmune disorder
- Reduces risk of MS and Cancer
- Reduces risk of influenza

VITAMIN A

Vitamin A is found in three main forms: retinol (Vitamin A1); 3, 4-didehydroretinol (Vitamin A2); and 3-hydroxy-retinol (Vitamin A3). Foods rich in vitamin A include liver, sweet potatoes, carrots, milk, egg yolks, and mozzarella cheese. Vitamin A is a group of nutritionally unsaturated hydrocarbons, which include retinol, retinal, retinoic acid, and several provitamin A carotenoids (beta, alpha, and gamma), among which beta-carotene is the most important. Vitamin A has multiple functions. It is important for growth and development, for the maintenance of the immune system, and good vision. The retinoids come from animals and fish. The carotenoids come from plants and are called provitamins (stored in the liver and converted into usable vitamin as needed).

Benefits of Vitamin A:

- Reduces risk of cancer
- Required for vision and healthy mucous membranes
- Strengthens bone development
- Important for growth and support of the skin
- Needed to detoxify PCB and dioxin
- Helps immune function (improves white blood cells, macrophages, natural killer cells, T and B lymphocytes

VITAMIN E

Vitamin E (alpha-tocopherol) is found in almonds, in many oils including wheat germ, safflower, corn, and soybean oils, and is also found in mangos, nuts, broccoli, and other foods. Vitamin E refers to a group of eight fat-soluble compounds that include both tocopherols (alpha, beta, gamma, and delta) and tocotrienols (alpha, beta, gamma, and delta). It's an antioxidant that comes as natural (d-alpha) and synthetic (dl-alpha). Of course, it is absorbed best by the body and metabolized by the liver in its natural form. D-alpha tocopherol is the most biologically active.

Benefits of Tocopherols in Your Body:

- Helps prevent Alzheimer's disease: lung, esophageal, and colorectal cancer
- Acts like estrogen and relieves hot flashes, decreases atrophic vaginitis, and helps ovarian function
- Inhibits platelet adhesion and prevents vascular damage from cholesterol-like substances
- Improves the action of insulin and helps your immune system
- Strengthens vitamin A and increase its storage

Benefits of Tocotrienols in Your Body:

- Decreases inflammation
- Lowers cholesterol
- Decreases risk of cancer
- Decreases plaque build-up

VITAMIN K

Vitamin K is fat-soluble and comes in two forms (K1 and K2). K1 is found in green leafy vegetables. K2 is formed from K1 and from friendly bacteria in the gastrointestinal tract.

Benefits of Vitamin K in Your Body:

- Enhances new bone growth
- Required in the synthesis of osteocalcin (helps in bone building)
- Improves clot formation
- Decreases calcium loss
- Helps bony mineralization
- Decreases calcification leading to decreased risk of coronary artery disease

WATER-SOLUBLE VITAMINS (B AND C)

There are 11 vitamins in the B complex. They work synergistically. Since they are eliminated from your body daily, they should be consumed multiple times per day. Supplementation with only B 12 can cause an imbalance in the other B vitamins.

B1 (thiamin) is needed for burning of carbohydrates for energy.

Benefits of B1 (Thiamin) in Your Body:

- Synthesis of nucleic acids and coenzymes
- Synthesis of aldosterone (water balancing hormone)
- Energy production (krebs cycle) and nerve function

- Metabolism of thyroid hormones and acetylcholine
- Enzyme activation in the adrenal glands
- Stress control and adrenal burnout

B2 (Riboflavin) is needed for energy production and tissue repair.

Benefits of B2 (Riboflavin) in Your Body:

- Converts vitamin B6, niacin, folic acid, and vitamin A to active form
- Assists in the regeneration of glutathione
- Energy metabolism and vitamin K
- Cytochrome P450 system
- Helps reactions that process carbs, fats, and proteins

B3 (Niacin and Niacinamide) is made from tryptophan, B6, B2, and iron. Niacin is used in over 40 chemical reactions in your body.

Benefits of B3 (Niacin) in Your Body:

- Function of the adrenal glands
- Assists in metabolism of carbohydrates, proteins, fats, tryptophan and seratonin
- Energy production, and conversion of cholesterol to pregnenolone
- Helps improve health of diabetics
- Lowers triglycerides and LDL and raises HDL
- Decreases lipoprotein A and fibrinogen

B5 (Pantothenic Acid) is primarily involved in metabolism of carbohydrates, fats, and protein.

Benefits of B5 (Pantothenic Acid) in Your Body:

- Synthesis of fatty acids, coenzyme A, and formation of antibodies
- Assists in red cell production and stimulates adrenal gland
- Helps your body use other vitamins and helps with fatty acid transport
- Helps in wound healing
- Helps convert food into energy
- Helps with synthesis of several amino acids
- Makes vitamin D

B6 (Pyridoxine) is a cofactor in many reactions of amino acid metabolism.

Benefits of B6 (Pyridoxine) in Your Body:

- Synthesis of hydrochloric acid and amino acids
- Assists in absorption of fats and protein
- Helps with the immune system and REM sleep
- Helps with synthesis of several neurotransmitters, serotonin and tryptophan
- Helps with methylation and detoxification
- Strengthening connective tissue

B7 (Biotin) is made by the gut flora and is involved in fat and protein metabolism. Increased stress and antibiotics destroys the gut flora and, hence, decreases biotin.

Benefits of B7 (Biotin) in Your Body:

- Energy production
- Assists in fatty acid metabolism
- Increases insulin sensitivity
- Strengthens nails

B9 (Folic Acid) is important for energy production and the immune system. The natural form is folate and the synthetic form is folic acid. Some of the folate is made in the intestines and the rest comes from food or supplements.

Benefits of B9 (Folic Acid) in Your Body:

- Metabolism of hemoglobin
- Assists in detoxification of hormones and phenol
- Essential for CNS function and DNA synthesis
- Helps with methylation
- Helps metabolic conversion of dopamine
- Helps with tissue health
- Protects baby from neural tube defects
- Produces SAMe and complex phospholipids for neurological function

B12 (Cobalamin) has a key role in the normal functioning of the brain and nervous system, and for the formation of blood. It is involved in the metabolism of every cell of the human body, especially affecting DNA synthesis and regulation, fatty acid synthesis, and energy production. Only bacteria and archaea have the enzymes required for its synthesis. Many foods are a natural source of B12 because of bacterial symbiosis.

Benefits of B12 (Cobalamin) in Your Body:

- Important for protein and DNA synthesis
- Assists in folic acid metabolism
- Essential for CNS function and proper digestion
- Helps with red blood cell metabolism
- Helps with carnitine and neurotransmitter metabolism
- Functions as a methyl donor

CHOLINE

Choline is the precursor molecule for the neurotransmitter acetylcholine, which is involved in many functions, including memory and muscle control. It is involved in almost every bodily system. Choline must be consumed through the diet for the body to remain healthy. It is used in the synthesis of the constructional components in the body's cell membranes.

Benefits of Choline in Your Body:

- Component of every cell membrane
- Assists in fat metabolism
- Essential for CNS function
- Helps with movement and coordination
- Precursor to acetylcholine
- Lowers LDL cholesterol

INOSITOL

Inositol helps synthesize phospholipids. It is essential for digestion, absorption, and transportation of fats in the body.

Benefits of Inositol in Your Body:

- Important for metabolism of estrogen and progesterone
- Assists in treatment of depression and panic disorder
- Involved in metabolism of fats and cholesterol
- Augments effects of neurotransmitter release
- Improves quality of sleep
- Protects arteries from hardening
- Reduces LDL cholesterol
- Has a calming effect
- Helps with lecithin formation

VITAMIN C

Vitamin C (ascorbic acid) can be found in high abundance in many fruits and vegetables and is also found in cereals, beef, poultry, and fish. Vitamin C is a cofactor in at least eight enzymatic reactions. It has to be consumed, because the body cannot make it. It is water-soluble and affects the immune system.

Benefits of Vitamin C in Your Body:

- Helps with wound healing and synthesis of collagen
- Assists the immune system by increasing white blood cells and interferons

- Decreases adrenal steroid and leukotrienes productions
- Decreases gum disease and stomach cancer
- Decreases risk of CAD
- Helps carnitine and tyrosine synthesis
- Is a powerful antioxidant
- Decreases blood pressure, incident of cataracts, and triglycerides
- Helps regenerate vitamin E, glutathione, and uric acid
- Increases fertility, HDL cholesterol, and nitric oxide
- Enhances iron absorption and progesterone production
- Helps with catecholamine and serotonin synthesis
- Prevents free radical damage of LDL
- Decreases lung disease, bruising, and damage due to glycation
- Helps mitochondria function
- Prevents formation of nitrosamines

MINERALS

A **mineral** is a naturally occurring substance that is solid and stable at room temperature. It is represented by a chemical formula, and has an ordered atomic structure. It is different from a rock, which can be an aggregate of minerals or non-minerals, and does not have a specific chemical composition. Our bodies cannot produce minerals. The amount of minerals required is based on diet, mineral content of the soil in which the food is grown, medications, health, age, and the interactions of the mineral with other substances.

There are two types of minerals; **macro,** of which we need large quantities; and **micro,** of which trace amounts are needed. Macro minerals (calcium, chloride, magnesium, phosphorus, potassium, and sodium) are needed in portions greater than 200 milligrams per day. Micro minerals (arsenic, boron, chromium, cobalt, copper, fluoride, iodine, iron, manganese, molybdenum, nickel, selenium, silicon, tin, vanadium, and zinc) require trace amounts less than 200 milligrams per day.

Organic (minerals from a living source—animal or plant) are much more readily absorbed into the body. Inorganic (not from living source) minerals are very poorly absorbed. It is important to find out if the vitamins or minerals you are taking are organic or inorganic.

RESVERATROL

Resveratrol is a stibenoid. It is a natural phenol and a phytoalexin produced naturally by several plants. It is extracted from the roots of the Japanese Knotweed when under attack by pathogens such as bacteria or fungi.

Resveratrol has been found to induce cell death when added to cancer cells grown in culture. Cancer cells grow rapidly and do not respond to cell death signals. Resveratrol has been found to inhibit proliferation (growth) and induce apoptosis (death) in a number of cancer cell lines.

Cancerous cells invade normal tissue aided by enzymes called matrix metalloproteinases. Resveratrol has been found to inhibit the activity of at least one type of matrix metalloproteinase. In order to grow rapidly, invasive tumors must develop new blood vessels by a process known as angiogenesis (blood vessel formation). Resveratrol has been found to inhibit angiogenesis.

Inflammation promotes cellular proliferation and angiogenesis and inhibits apoptosis. Resveratrol has been found to inhibit the activity of several inflammatory enzymes, including cyclooxygenase and lipoxygenase. Resveratrol may also inhibit pro-inflammatory transcription factors, such as Nuclear factor kappaB (NFκB) or Activator protein (AP).

Atherosclerosis is now recognized as an inflammatory disease, and several measures of inflammation are associated with increased risk of myocardial infarction (heart attack). One of the earliest events in the development of atherosclerosis is the recruitment of inflammatory white blood cells from the blood to the arterial wall by vascular cell adhesion molecules. Resveratrol has been found to inhibit the expression of adhesion molecules in cultured endothelial cells.

The proliferation of vascular smooth muscle cells plays an important role in the progression of atherosclerosis. Resveratrol has been found to inhibit the proliferation of vascular smooth muscle cells in culture.

Endothelial Nitric Oxide Synthase (eNOS) Activity is an enzyme that catalyzes the formation of nitric oxide (NO) by vascular endothelial cells. NO is needed to maintain arterial relaxation (vasodilation), and impaired NO-dependent vasodilation is associated with increased risk of cardiovascular disease. Resveratrol has been found to stimulate eNOS activity in cultured endothelial cells.

Platelet aggregation is one of the first steps in the formation of a blood clot that can occlude a coronary or cerebral artery, resulting in myocardial infarction or stroke. Resveratrol has been found to inhibit platelet aggregation.

Resveratrol has been found to exert a number of potentially cardioprotective effects, including inhibition of platelet aggregation. promotion of vasodilation by enhancing the production of NO, and inhibition of inflammatory enzymes. The concentrations of resveratrol required to produce these effects are often higher than those that have been measured in human plasma after oral consumption of resveratrol. The results of some animal studies suggest that high oral doses of resveratrol could decrease the risk of thrombosis (clot formation) and atherosclerosis. One study found increased atherosclerosis in animals fed resveratrol. Although its presence in red wine has stimulated a great deal of interest in the potential for resveratrol to prevent cardiovascular disease, there is currently no convincing evidence that resveratrol has cardio-protective effects in humans, particularly in the amounts present in 1–2 glasses of red wine.

Resveratrol has been found to inhibit the proliferation of a variety of human cancer cell lines, including those from breast, prostate, stomach, colon, pancreatic, and thyroid cancers. In animal models, oral administration of resveratrol inhibited the development of esophageal, intestinal, and breast cancer (two induced by chemical carcinogens). Oral resveratrol was not effective in inhibiting the development of lung cancer induced by carcinogens in cigarette smoke.

GLUTHATIONE

Glutathione is a tripetide (composed of three amino acids—cysteine, glutamic acid, and glycine). It is found in every cell and is responsible for the health of the cell. It is an antioxidant that prevents damage to the cell by reactive oxygen species, such as free radicals and peroxides. Levels of gluthatione begin to diminish at about 40 years of age. Glutathione occurs naturally in many foods, such as fresh fruits and vegetables. It protects against aging, cancer, heart disease, dementia, autism, Alzheimer's, and numerous other medical problems.

Poor diet, pollution, toxins, stress, medication, trauma, aging, infections, and radiation deplete gluthathione. This leaves you susceptible to unrestrained cell disintegration from oxidative stress, free radicals, infections, and cancer. Furthermore, your liver gets overloaded and damaged, making it unable to do its job of detoxification.

Benefits of Glutathione in Your Body:

- Enhances liver and brain detoxification of toxic chemicals and heavy metals
- Helps to recycle other antioxidants, like vitamin C and E
- Involved in protein and prostaglandin synthesis
- Is a neuromodulator (transmit information between neurons)
- It is the major endogenous antioxidant produced by the cells
- Decreases sugar cravings
- Is a neurotransmitter
- Helps regulate your immune system
- Is used in DNA synthesis and repair, amino acid transport, and enzyme activation
- Is a very powerful antioxidant

ANTIOXIDANTS

An **antioxidant** is a molecule that inhibits the oxidation of other molecules. Oxidation is a chemical reaction that transfers electrons or hydrogen from a substance to an oxidizing agent. Oxidation reactions can produce free radicals. In turn, these radicals can start chain reactions. When the chain reaction occurs in a cell, it can cause damage or death to the cell. Antioxidants terminate these chain reactions by removing free radical intermediates, and inhibit other oxidation reactions. They do this by being oxidized themselves.

Antioxidants protect your cells against the effects of free radicals. Free radicals are produced when your body breaks down food, or by environmental exposures, such as tobacco smoke and radiation. Free radicals can damage cells, and may play a role in heart disease, cancer, and other diseases. Antioxidants are found in many foods. These include fruits and vegetables, nuts, grains, and some meats, poultry, and fish.

EXAMPLES OF ANTIOXIDANTS:

- **Beta-carotene** is found in many foods that are orange in color, including sweet potatoes, carrots, cantaloupe, squash, apricots, pumpkin, and mangos. Some green, leafy vegetables, including collard greens, spinach, and kale, are also rich in beta-carotene.

- **Lutein** is best known for its association with healthy eyes, and is abundant in green, leafy vegetables such as collard greens, spinach, and kale

- **Lycopene** is a potent antioxidant found in tomatoes, watermelon, guava, papaya, apricots, pink grapefruit, blood oranges, and other foods. Approximately 85 percent of American dietary intake of lycopene comes from tomatoes and tomato products.

- **Selenium** is a mineral. Foods such as rice and wheat are the major dietary sources of selenium. The amount of selenium in soil determines the amount of selenium in the foods grown in that soil. Animals that eat grains or plants grown in selenium-rich soil have higher levels of selenium in their muscle. In the United States, meats and bread are common sources of dietary selenium. Brazil nuts also contain large quantities of selenium.

Foods High in Antioxidants

Corn	Carrots	Acai Berry
Lime	Oregano	Pinto Beans
Kale	Spinach	Broad Beans
Lemon	Apricots	Wheat Germ
Dates	Broccoli	Hempseed Oil
Chiles	Cinnamon	Barley & Rye
Cloves	Tomatoes	Black Currant
Garlic	Artichoke	Blood Oranges
Grapes	Green Tea	Sweet Potatoes
Prunes	Pineapple	Raw Nuts & Seeds
Mangos	Red Beets	Whole Grain Brown Rice
Squash	Pomegranates	Coconut Oil
Millet	Peppers	Goji Berries
Almonds	Olive Oil	Berries

ENZYME THERAPY

At any given moment, enzymes are doing all of the work being done inside any cell. A bacterium like E. coli has about 1,000 different types of enzymes floating around in the cytoplasm at any given time. Enzymes are little chemical-reaction machines. They are highly selective catalysis, greatly accelerating both the rate and specificity of metabolic reactions, from the digestion of food to the synthesis of DNA.

Almost all chemical reactions in a biological cell need enzymes in order to occur at rates sufficient for life. The purpose of an enzyme in a cell is to allow the cell to carry out chemical reactions very quickly. These reactions allow the cell to build things or take things apart as needed. This is how a cell grows and reproduces.

Enzymes are proteins made from amino acids. An enzyme encompasses 100 to 1,000 amino acids in a very specific and unique order. The chain of amino acids then folds into a unique shape. That shape allows the enzyme to carry out specific chemical reactions. An enzyme acts as a very efficient catalyst for a specific chemical reaction. The enzyme speeds that reaction up tremendously.

The sugar maltose is made from two glucose molecules bonded together. The enzyme maltase is shaped in such a way that it can break the bond and free the two glucose pieces. The only thing maltase can do is break maltose molecules, but it can do that very rapidly and efficiently. Other types of enzymes can put atoms and molecules together. Breaking molecules apart and putting molecules together is what enzymes do. There is a specific enzyme for each chemical reaction needed to make the cell work properly.

In people who are lactose intolerant, the sugar in milk (lactose) does not get broken into its glucose components. Therefore, it cannot be digested. The intestinal cells of lactose intolerant people do not produce lactase, the enzyme needed to break down lactose. This problem shows how the lack of just one enzyme in the human body can lead to problems. A person who is lactose intolerant can swallow a drop of lactase prior to drinking milk and the problem is solved.

Within a bacterium, there are thousands of enzymes (lactase being one of them). All of the enzymes float freely in the cytoplasm waiting for the chemical they recognize to float by. There are hundreds or millions of copies of each different type of enzyme, depending on how important a reaction is to a cell and how often the reaction is needed. These enzymes do everything from breaking glucose down for energy to building cell walls, constructing new enzymes, and allowing the cell to reproduce. Enzymes do all of the work inside cells.

Biochemical reactions in living organisms are essentially energy transfers. Often, they occur together as oxidation/reduction reactions. Reduction is the gain of an electron. Oxidation is the loss of an electron. In oxidation/reduction reactions, one chemical is oxidized, and its electrons are passed to another (reduced) chemical.

Vitamin, minerals, and enzymes are the tools of your body. **Nothing** is made or broken down by your body without its tools. There are millions of chemical reactions taking place in your body every second. They all require the tools to make them happen. The water-soluble minerals have to be replaced on a daily basis. As we age, our ability to obtain and use vitamin, minerals and enzymes decreases. We need to actively supplement our diet with all three as we age to remain young and healthy.

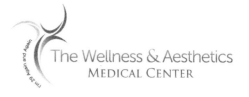

Chapter Six

ENVIRONMENTAL ALLERGY & FOOD SENSITIVITIES CONTROL

ENVIRONMENTAL ALLERGIES

One out of five Americans suffer from allergies. For some, allergies are simply a short-lived nuisance; however, for millions, it's a life-altering disease. Because many allergic reactions are not identifiable as such, allergies may go unnoticed and untreated for the majority of a person's life.

Allergies occur when the body's immune system overreacts to particles that are normally harmless. In environmental allergies, the body's immune system overreacts to allergens from animals and dust mites, or pollens from grasses, weeds, trees, and molds that are present in the air that you breathe. When these allergens enter the nose, sinuses, and lungs, the body's immune system overreacts to these particles and releases a number of chemicals, including histamine and leukotrienes (inflammatory mediators), resulting in what are called allergic reactions.

Symptoms of environmental allergies (allergic rhinitis)

- Sneezing
- Runny nose—usually the drainage is clear and watery
- Stuffy nose
- Itchy nose
- Post-nasal drip
- Itchy or scratchy throat
- Sinus pain or pressure
- Itchy eyes
- Watery eyes
- Red puffy eyes

Exposure to allergens can lead to an immediate reaction, or the reaction can be delayed. Symptoms can also be seasonal. Individuals with environmental allergies also can develop frequent ear or sinus infections, difficulties sleeping, snoring, fatigue, depression, and decreased attention span. They are also at increased risk of developing asthma and atopic dermatitis (eczema).

The only reliable treatment for allergies is immunotherapy, which involves gradual delivery of the substances that trigger allergies to acclimate the body to the world around it. Treating the underlying cause is the focus of sublingual (oral drops) immunotherapy, compared to over-the-counter and prescription drugs, which provide relief from symptoms but do nothing to cure the underlying problem.

FOOD ALLERGIES OR FOOD INTOLERANCES

Food allergies or food intolerances affect nearly everyone at some point. One out of three people has a food allergy. A food allergy, or hypersensitivity, is an abnormal response to a food, triggered by the immune system. Even though the immune system is responsible for food allergies it is not the cause of symptoms of food intolerance.

Food allergies involve two features of the human immune response. One is the production of immunoglobulin E (IgE), an antibody that circulates through the blood. The other is the mast cell, a cell that occurs in all body tissues. It is common in areas of the body that are typical sites of allergic reactions (nose, throat, lungs, skin, and gastrointestinal tract).

A person who is predisposed to form IgE to foods first has to be exposed to the food. When this food is digested, it triggers certain cells to produce specific IgE in large amounts. The IgE is then released and attaches to the surface of mast cells. The next time the person eats that food, it interacts with specific IgE on the surface of the mast cells and triggers the cells to release chemicals, such as histamine. Depending upon the tissue in which they are released, these chemicals will cause a person to have various food allergy symptoms. If the mast cells release chemicals in the ears, nose, and throat, a person may feel an itching in the mouth and may have difficulty breathing or swallowing. If the affected mast cells are in the gastrointestinal tract, the person may have abdominal pain, bloating, vomiting, or diarrhea. The chemicals released by skin mast cells can cause hives.

More than 140 different foods have been identified as causes of allergic reactions. According to a recent report by the U.S. Centers for Disease Control, 90 percent of food allergies are associated with eight food types:

- Cow's milk
- Hen's eggs
- Peanuts
- Soy foods
- Wheat
- Fish
- Crustacean shellfish (such shrimp, prawns, lobster, and crab)
- Tree nuts (such as almonds, cashews, walnuts, pecans, pistachios, Brazil nuts, hazelnuts, and chestnuts)

Foods that are least often associated with any type of food allergy include:

- Apples
- Lamb
- Pears
- Winter Squash
- Sweet Potatoes
- Cherries
- Carrots
- Rice

FOOD SENSITIVITIES

Compared to food allergies, food sensitivities are more common and have a wider and more varied impact on our health. Food sensitivities also include food intolerances, which, unlike allergies, are toxic reactions to foods that do not involve the immune system and are often more difficult to diagnose. Some of the symptoms of food sensitivities including bloating, abdominal pain, vomiting, diarrhea, blood in the stool, eczema, urticaria (hives), skin rashes, wheezing, and runny noses. Food sensitivities may also cause fatigue, gas, mood swings, nervousness, migraines, eating disorders, and many other conditions. These symptoms, which are more commonly related to food intolerance, are less often associated with the consumption of food.

Some foods can cause inflammation in people who are sensitive to them. Some anti-inflammatory foods and herbs are ginger, curcumin, rosemary, basil, and cherries.

Food allergies and leaky gut

Inflammation and stress can cause "leaky gut" (the condition when your small intestinal wall is broken down, allowing large food particles to pass through). Leaky gut can be caused by intestinal inflammations from parasite or microbial infections, as well as by a food allergy response, and can result in the development of multiple food allergies. Left untreated, inflammation of the intestinal wall caused by allergic reactions to one food can facilitate allergic responses to other foods, because the inflamed wall of the intestine allows toxic food molecules into the body that normally would be prevented from entering. Food allergy responses tax the ability of the macrophages to eliminate damaging food molecules. The immune system gets overwhelmed and increasing numbers of toxic food molecules are allowed into the body.

Leaky gut can often prevent the absorption of nutrients vital to your health. Nutrients are normally absorbed through the cells at the tip of the intestinal villi. When the intestine is damaged from inflammation, the villi are no longer healthy and intact. The intestine is unable to properly absorb the available nutrients. Cow's milk, eggs, soy, and wheat are common allergens that are associated with intestinal inflammation and leaky gut.

Leaky gut can lead to autoimmune diseases like Diabetes (DM) Hashimoto thyroiditis, Irritable Bowel Syndrome (IBS), Crohn's disease, joint and muscle pain, depression, obesity, hormone imbalance, and numerous other medical conditions.

FOOD INTOLERANCES

There are many types of food intolerances. The most common are intolerances to:

- Lactose (affects 10 percent of adults)
- Tyrosine
- Preservatives and Additives
- Gluten

We crave the foods we are most allergic or sensitive to. Succumbing to food cravings to help alleviate symptoms is the beginning of a cycle of short-term relief from symptoms and craving of the food, as symptoms will increase again. This yo-yo effect is believed by some allergy specialists to be the reason why people who stop eating the foods to which they are allergic (go on elimination or avoidance diets) first go through several days when they feel worse before they start feeling much better.

The elimination diet

The allergy avoidance diet (the elimination diet) is instrumental in avoiding allergic reactions to food and is the way to break the cycle of addiction. The elimination diet allows the body to completely remove the antigen providing no reason for the formation of antibodies. As a result, some people can go back to eating a food to which they were once allergic after a year or two of avoiding the food.

A person will experience more symptoms for the first several days to a week when first beginning the elimination diet. Some believe this is caused by the cross-linking of antibodies, while others believe it is because the body is starting to mobilize toxins that had been stored in fat tissue and other storage sites in the body. It is important to remain on the elimination diet even if symptoms appear to be increasing. After staying on the diet for several weeks, you should begin to feel relief from symptoms and generally feel much better.

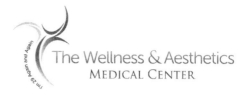
Chapter Seven

NEUROTRANSMITTERS AND THE NEURO-ENDO-IMMUNE (NEI) SUPER-SYSTEM

We've talked about imbalances in our nutrition and in our hormones, and how they can wreak havoc with our well-being. Now, let's delve into a lesser known, but equally important, topic in our wellness: correcting imbalance in our neurotransmitters.

We all have heard about hormones. Neurotransmitters are the hormones of the brain. Neurotransmitter imbalances are at the foundation of many psychiatric and neurological disorders. Imbalances in neurotransmission, due to excessive or deficient neurotransmitter levels are associated with depression, insomnia, anxiety, behavioral disorders, memory disorders, and a spectrum of other brain-related functions. Because neurotransmitters play an integral role in these disease states, they are prime targets for treating disorders of the nervous system and mental health concerns.

External interventions from pharmaceutical medications or nutritional supplements can alter nervous system function. Pharmaceutical medications influence neurotransmission, while nutritional neuromodulators (amino acids, standardized herbal extracts, vitamins and minerals, and phospholipid derivatives) utilize dietary constituents and naturally derived substances to influence neurotransmission.

Pharmaceutical and nutritional neuromodulators can be classified based on their function in the nervous system.

FIVE CLASSES OF NEUROMODULATORS INCLUDE:

- Reuptake inhibitors
- Enzyme modulators
- Receptor modifiers
- Enzymatic cofactors
- Neurotransmitter substrates

How do neurotransmitters work?

Our nervous system is comprised of a network of specialized cells, called neurons. Information is relayed by neurons using electrical and chemical signals. Neurons are composed of two primary structures: dendrites and axons. Dendrites receive messages from other neurons. Axons send messages via electrical signals and the release of chemicals called neurotransmitters. The neurotransmitters are released into the space between adjacent neurons. The space between neurons is called the synapse.

The axon is a hair-like extension of the cytoplasm of the neuron. The axon is wrapped in a myelin sheath that serves to insulate the electrical messages passing through it. The neurotransmitter molecules are stored in vesicles within the axon terminals. The vesicles are translocated along the axon and released at the nerve terminal when the neuron is activated.

The nervous system is the primary communication system in the body. Structurally, it is divided into the central nervous system and the peripheral nervous system. The central nervous system consists of the brain and spinal cord, while the peripheral nervous system is present throughout the rest of the body, linking the brain to the organs, tissues, and glands, through the spinal cord. Functionally, the nervous system can be divided between the somatic nervous system and the autonomic nervous system. The somatic nervous system is responsible for coordinating muscle and body movements and receiving external stimuli. The autonomic nervous system maintains internal balance or homeostasis within the body and can be further divided into the sympathetic and parasympathetic divisions.

The sympathetic division is responsible for the "flight or fight" response. It mobilizes energy stores, increases cardiac output, and dilates bronchial passages. The primary messengers of this system are acetylcholine, epinephrine, and norepinephrine.

The parasympathetic division of the autonomic nervous system conserves energy and increases intestinal and glandular activity. The primary messenger is acetylcholine.

NEI

The Neuro-Endo-Immune (NEI) Super-system incorporates three vital disciplines: Neurology, Endocrinology, and Immunology. Evaluation of the NEI Super-system (through the measurement of neurotransmitters, hormones, and cytokines) represents nervous, endocrine, and immune function, respectively. Assessment of these essential biochemical mediators provides important insight into the root causes contributing to clinical conditions.

Neuroendoimmunology is an emerging field of medical science that seeks to understand the interconnectedness of the nervous, endocrine, and immune systems. Progressive research in this field suggests each of these three systems function as a larger whole, termed the "NEI Supersystem." Within this supersystem, the nervous system plays the integral role of modulating the function of the immune and endocrine systems via the hypothalamic–pituitary axes and innervations of endocrine and immunological organs.

Due to the interconnected nature of this larger system, the effects of the endocrine and immune systems also reciprocally influence the nervous system. Disruptions in the function of one system will ultimately have an impact on the function of all three systems.

An emotion is the psychophysiological response to the interactions between biochemical and environmental stimuli. Many expressed emotions have been shown to stimulate specific brain regions. This stimulation is biochemical in nature involving the release of neurotransmitters. Reinforcement, from continual stimulation, leads to the strengthening of neurocircuit patterns and results in learned behavior. Neuroplasticity is the ability to add or change neuroncircuitry to allow for adaptation, learning, and general health.

Neuroplasticity is biochemical and is a direct result of neural membrane health, neurotransmitter levels, and receptor viability. It is influenced by the immune system, chronic inflammation, and mental thoughts. Mental and emotional therapies for behavioral modifications are directly supported when the biochemistry of neuroplasticity is also addressed.

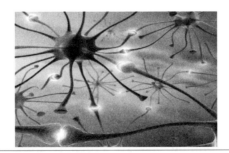

THE IMPACT OF CHRONIC STRESS

Chronic stress is the result of prolonged response to a perceived burden. Microglia are the macrophages of the central nervous system (CNS). They release pro-inflammatory cytokines (TNF-α and IL-1) during an immune response. TNF-α and IL-1 induce the enzyme indolamine dioxygenase (IDO). This promotes the conversion of tryptophan to quinolinic acid. Quinolinic acid stimulates glutamate receptors, which could enhance a stress response. Emotional stress can trigger the HPA axis and the release of cortisol. This tends to inhibit pro-inflammatory and support anti-inflammatory mediators. Under chronic stress, the cortisol response can become blunted, which could prevent the body's ability to keep inflammation under control.

Neurotransmitter imbalances associated with psychiatric complaints can both arise from and cause imbalances in the immune and endocrine systems. Increasing IDO can indirectly suppress serotonin production by promoting tryptophan (the precursor of serotonin) conversion down the kynurenine pathway. Serotonin triggers mast cell migration to the site of injury. Estradiol can bind to and activate the serotonin receptor, which may partly explain mood changes during menopause.

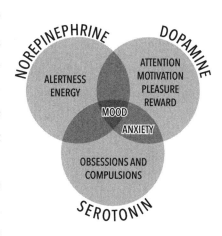

Estradiol and serotonin

At optimal levels, estradiol (E2) supports serotonin in several ways:

- E2 increases tryptophan hydroxylase, the rate-limiting step in serotonin synthesis

- E2 receptor (E2β) simulation up-regulates the expression of serotonin receptors (5-HT2A)

- E2 acts as a serotonin reuptake inhibitor

- E2 inhibits monoamine oxidase activity, thus preventing the breakdown of serotonin

Consequently, if estradiol levels decrease, serotonin activity may decrease as well. Low estradiol levels may result in symptoms associated with low serotonin (e.g., low mood, sleep difficulties, hot flashes, uncontrolled appetite, and headaches). Supporting serotonin may counter the effects of decreased estradiol.

Progesterone and GABA

Progesterone's metabolite allopregnanolone acts at the GABA receptor to increase GABA activity, thus promoting calming effects. Low progesterone levels may result in symptoms associated with low GABA (e.g., anxiousness and sleep difficulties). Supporting GABA may counter the effects of decreased progesterone.

Cortisol and the monoamines

Cortisol can stimulate monoamine oxidase (MAO) to dampen the production of various neurotransmitters, including serotonin, epinephrine, norepinepherine, and dopamine. MAO can enhance tyrosine hydroxylase to cause an increase in the same neurotransmitters, including GABA. An up-regulated immune system can be dampened by increased cortisol.

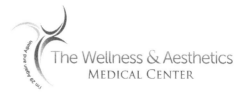
Chapter Eight

GROWING YOUNGER

N ow that our systems are in balance and we are feeling younger, we're ready to start talking about growing younger. At the Wellness and Aesthetics Medical Center, we help people grow younger every day. I consider myself the ringleader. We are always searching for the fountain of youth.

In order to understand what "growing younger" really means, let's begin by looking at what causes us to age, and how it can be stopped and even reversed; the process of **telomerase activation.**

TELOMERASE ACTIVATION

Telomeres are sections of genetic material at the end of each chromosome whose primary function is to prevent chromosomal "fraying" when a cell replicates. As a cell ages, its telomeres become shorter. Eventually, the telomeres become too short to allow cell replication, the cell stops dividing and will ultimately die; a normal biological process.

Age-adjusted telomere length is currently one of the best methods to assess biological age, using structural analysis of chromosomal change in the telomere. Serial evaluation of telomere length is an indicator of how rapidly one ages relative to a normal population.

Therapies directed at slowing the loss of telomere length may slow aging and age-related diseases.

There are over 100 trillion cells in our body, and at any given time a great number are dividing to keep us alive. The process is propagated by genes sitting on the 23 pairs of chromosomes found in the nucleus of each cell. The chromosomes are long sequences of DNA that contain all our genetic material. Each pair of chromosomes consists of one from your mother and one from your father, and they are twisted around each other to form a structure called the "double helix."

Telomeres have no genetic function. They are simply stretches of DNA (repeats of base pairs) that protect the rest of the chromosome. These little bits of DNA are critical to healthy cell function and have been likened to the plastic tips on shoelaces, because they prevent the chromosome from "fraying."

Each time the cell divides, the telomeres become progressively shorter. When they get too short, the cells reach replicative senescence (cell death) and can no longer divide. This leads to conditions associated with old age. We have only recently begun to understand the critical importance of shortened telomeres. People over 60 who have long telomeres experience greater heart and immune system health than do their age-matched counterparts with shorter telomeres.

It is well understood that maintaining telomere length is an important way of preventing age-related decline. Professor Lenhard Hayflick first noted the phenomenon of cellular aging in 1961. He discovered that cells couldn't divide beyond a specific number of times. This is called the Hayflick Limit. Cells reaching this limit become old. Professor Hayflick had no idea what caused it. The role telomeres play in cellular aging was finally understood in 1990. Calvin Harley at McMaster University in Canada and Carol Greider at Cold Spring Harbor Laboratory in the United States discovered that telomere shortening goes hand-in-hand with the aging process. Cells reaching the Hayflick Limit were caused by telomere shortening.

We've already talked about the many illnesses that inflammation can create. An inflammatory diet (one that increases oxidative stress) will also shorten telomeres faster. This includes refined carbohydrates, fast foods, processed foods, sodas, artificial sweeteners, trans fats, and saturated fats. Conversely, a diet with a large amount and variety of antioxidants that improves oxidative defense and reduces oxidative stress will slow telomere shortening. Consumption of 10 servings of fresh and relatively uncooked fruits and vegetables, mixed fiber, monounsaturated fats, omega-3 fatty acids, cold-water fish, and high-quality vegetable proteins will help preserve telomere length. We advise reducing total daily caloric intake and implementing an exercise program. Fasting for 12 hours each night at least four days per week will help, too.

Lifestyle modifications, like achieving ideal body weight and body composition with low body fat (less than 22 percent for women and less than 16 percent for men), are also helpful. Decreasing visceral fat is very important. Regular aerobic and resistance exercise for at least one hour per day, sleeping for at least eight hours each night, and stress reduction, along with discontinuation of the use of all tobacco products, are strongly recommended. Bioidentical hormone replacement therapy may decrease the rate of telomere loss, too.

Testing should be done once a year to evaluate the rate of aging and to make adjustments in nutrition, nutritional supplements, weight management, exercise, and other lifestyle modifications known to influence telomere length.

Oxidative stress will shorten telomere length and cause aging in cellular tissue. Antioxidant supplements can reduce oxidative stress, improve oxidative defenses and mitochondrial function, reduce inflammation, and slow vascular aging. Supplementation is very important. Antioxidants work synergistically and must be balanced to work most effectively.

Increasing antioxidant capacity at the cellular level is critical to maintaining telomere length. Recent evidence suggests that a high-quality and balanced multivitamin will also help maintain telomere length. Studies have linked longer telomeres with levels of vitamin E, vitamin C, vitamin D, omega-3 fatty acids, and the antioxidant resveratrol. Homocysteine levels have been inversely associated with telomere length, suggesting that reducing homocysteine levels via folate and vitamin B supplementation may decrease the rate of telomere loss.

Conditions such as cardiovascular disease, insulin resistance diabetes, hypertension, atherosclerosis, and dementia affect telomere length. Correcting subclinical nutritional deficiencies that may contribute to such diseases is crucial for telomere maintenance.

Some practitioners have recommended reducing coronary risk factors, inflammation, and oxidative stress levels to improve telomere length. Therapy should increase nitric oxide levels and nitric oxide bioavailability, increase arginine, increase endothelial progenitor cells (stem cells), improve mitochondrial function, and increase oxidative defenses. One should optimize hormone levels, exercise, sleep, nutrition, and nutritional supplements. Fasting and caloric restriction should be part of the regimen, as well.

Telomerase activation works on targeted cells in your body and can improve not only cell longevity but also quality of life. A double-blind, placebo controlled study of TA-65® showed improvements in:

- Immune system

- Vision

- Male sexual performance

- Skin appearance

You can learn more about telomerase activation as a method to intervene in the aging process at the Wellness and Aesthetics Medical Center. Understand how taking TA-65™ may improve your health and vitality. Find out your real biological age by testing your biomarkers of aging and measuring the length of your telomeres.

TA-65 is a naturally occurring single molecule found in the ancient Chinese herb astragalus. T.A. Sciences has developed a proprietary process to refine and purify TA-65. Their process begins with tons of plant material harvested from selected farms in one small region in China. In the plant extraction facility, the raw astragalus root is chopped up and refined. After initial extraction, the base ingredient is further purified and then sent to an outside government testing facility, where it is tested for purity, heavy metals, and pesticides. The product is then sent to an FDA-certified, state-of-the-art laboratory for final purification that ends up with 90+ percent pure TA-65.

Now, let's look at some of the other actions we can take toward regaining our youthful looks and feeling.

CELL-ASSISTED AUTOLOGOUS FAT-TRANSFER

Cell-assisted autologous fat transfer is a procedure in which a patient's own fat is used to augment sunken or thin regions of the face or body in order to add volume where it is desired. This procedure is a safe and scientifically proven process in which fat cells are harvested and redistributed to other areas of the body, most often to breasts and buttocks, or to the face, to eliminate wrinkles and facial drooping. This type of fat transfer has such applications as:

- Filling in forehead wrinkles and laugh lines
- Filling sunken areas under the eyes
- Cheek or chin augmentation
- Smoothing lines in the face
- Breast augmentation or reconstruction
- Gluteal (buttock) augmentation
- Improve facial or breast symmetry
- Lip augmentation

With cell-assisted autologous fat-transfer, a majority of the transferred fat remains in its place permanently. This leads to long-lasting results and fewer visits to the office. There is also very little risk for post-procedure complications.

Even though it may sound complex, autologous fat transfer is a simple procedure, requiring just five steps:

1. Excess fat from abdomen, buttocks, or thighs are removed.
2. Fat cells are isolated and cleansed.
3. Stem cells are extracted from a portion of the fat.
4. PRP is extracted from your blood.
5. The fat cells are then mixed with the stem cells and PRP and injected into the specified facial or body areas.

HYPERBARIC THERAPY

Hyperbaric oxygen therapy (HBOT) is a treatment modality where a patient breathes 100 percent oxygen while inside a treatment chamber at a pressure higher than sea level. This helps dissolve more oxygen in blood cells, plasma, and body fluids. The red blood cells (RBC) deliver more oxygen to the tissues and organs than do white blood cells (WBC), and WBCs perform more effectively. Increasing the person's oxygen levels allows the body to repair itself more effectively, promoting health and wellness. This therapeutic modality can be used to ameliorate a broad range of conditions in which oxygen breathed under increased atmospheric pressure can speed up wound healing and recovery.

Oxygen helps boost the health of every cell and helps the healing process. After any cosmetic surgery procedure, there is tissue that has undergone some trauma. If enough oxygen cannot reach these damaged areas, the healing time slows down. The use of HBOT in aesthetics therapies has increased. HBOT promotes enhanced collagen production, fibroblast proliferation, and neovascularization that support quicker granulation tissue formation and faster healing. Saturated levels of 100 percent oxygen in the bloodstream as well as all body fluids accelerate the formation of new capillary and peripheral blood vessels. This results in an effective and accelerated postoperative healing, with better aesthetic results. Post-operative recovery in junction with HBOT may make the healing process last for days instead of weeks, with less tissue trauma and a remarkable reduction of swelling, bruising, and a substantial control of possible infections.

Office cosmetic procedures and surgeries can all benefit from HBOT. These may include pre- and post-cosmetic intervention. This quickens the recovery process, with better aesthetic effects. HBOT also helps because of the anti-aging effects of hyperbaric pure oxygen. HBOT can increase circulating stem cells eight-fold.

NITRIC OXIDE (NO)

Nitric oxide, derived from arginine (an amino acid found in protein), is implicated in practically every cellular response and health condition imaginable, from the cardiovascular system to the immune system, and hormone function to nerve function. The following are the primary scientifically backed reasons why anyone should consider using high dose arginine to increase NO.

1. NO is 1,000 times more powerful than any naturally occurring antioxidant in the body. Its antioxidant properties support various body systems and may protect against heart disease, stroke, cancer, and diabetes, as well as slowing premature aging.

2. It offers wide-ranging cardiovascular support, including controlling blood pressure and plaque formation. Nitric oxide keeps arteries relaxed and pliable for normal blood pressure, preventing hypertension and angina.

3. It enhances memory, particularly long-term memories, and may help to reverse the effects of dementia and Alzheimer's disease.

4. It boosts human growth hormone (HGH) production, which has anti-aging properties.

5. It enhances communication of messenger cells between nerves and the brain.

6. It may help improve immune function and fight bacterial infections.

7. It may help in the treatment and prevention of diabetes and its complications, such as poor circulation and blindness. Arginine is also found to regulate insulin secretion in the pancreas.

8. It may inhibit the division and proliferation of cancer cells.

9. It helps with cholesterol control by lowering serum and LDL cholesterol levels.

10. It enhances male sexual performance by decreasing vascular erectile dysfunction.

11. Its anticoagulant abilities reduce clotting to lower heart attack and stroke risk.

12. It reduces pregnancy-related hypertension, a risk factor for both the expectant mother and the unborn child.

13. It is useful in the treatment of asthma by opening pulmonary pathways for easier breathing and the treatment of lung disorders.

14. It relaxes hypertonic sphincter muscles, preventing and healing hemorrhoids.

15. It boosts lean muscle mass and preserves bone density by increasing HGH production, which also leads to a reduction in fatty tissue. Because of these properties, it may be useful in weight management and strength training.

16. It can help offset cardiovascular and lung damage caused by tobacco use, since nitric oxide levels in smokers are less than half of those found in nonsmokers.

17. It helps to accelerate wound healing and postsurgery recovery. Research has shown it is useful in reducing burn wounds and stimulates wound healing in the elderly.

18. It may be useful in enhancing athletic performance due to its ability to boost exercise tolerance, its beneficial effect on the lungs, and its effect on HGH levels. This helps with building lean muscle tissue.

19. It may be used to improve the function of the prostate.

20. It may prevent and possibly reverse the effects of osteoporosis by positively affecting bone mass.

21. It has been used in the treatment of irritable bowel syndrome and to reduce the occurrence of ulcers—especially stress related—without affecting gastric acid production.

22. It may improve renal function and slow the progression of renal disease and age-related chronic renal failure. Arginine's protective effect on the kidneys may also benefit those with diabetes

Benefits of High-Dose L-Arginine:

- Supports cardiovascular health
- Enhances blood flow to vital organs
- Combats the negative effects of premature cardiovascular aging
- May aid in decreasing body fat
- Anti-aging benefits
- Supports healthy sexual performance

- □ Maintains healthy blood sugar levels already in normal range

- □ May boost energy levels

- □ Reduces arterial inflammation and oxidative stress

- □ Inhibits blood clots and lowers blood pressure

- □ Decreases stroke and heart disease

BETTER SLEEP

Poor sleep is a threat to your health. Harvard Medical School reports that sleep disorders and heart trouble go hand in hand. Poor sleep increases levels of CRP (inflammation). Sleep plays a critical role in immune function, metabolism, memory, learning, and other vital functions. One of the primary functions of sleep is to help organisms conserve their energy resources.

Both eating and sleeping are regulated by powerful internal drives. Going without food produces the uncomfortable sensation of hunger, while going without sleep makes us feel overwhelmingly fatigued. Just as eating relieves hunger and ensures that we obtain the nutrients we need, sleeping relieves sleepiness and ensures that we obtain the sleep we need.

Some providers believe sleep serves to "restore" what is lost in the body while we are awake. Sleep provides an opportunity for the body to repair and rejuvenate itself. The most striking evidence of this is provided by research that shows that animals deprived entirely of sleep lose all immune function and die in just a matter of weeks. This is further supported by findings that many of the major restorative functions in the body, like muscle growth, tissue repair, protein synthesis, and growth hormone release, occur mostly during sleep.

Other rejuvenating aspects of sleep are specific to the brain and cognitive functions. While we are awake, neurons in the brain produce adenosine, a by-product of the cells' activities. The build-up of adenosine in the brain is thought to be one factor that leads to our perception of being tired. Scientists think that this build-up of adenosine during wakefulness may promote the "drive to sleep." As long as we are awake, adenosine accumulates and remains high. During sleep, the body has a chance to clear adenosine from the system. As a result, we feel more alert when we are awake. Sleep plays a critical role in brain development in infants and young children. Infants spend about 13 to 14 hours per day sleeping, and about half of that time is spent in REM sleep, the stage in which most dreams occur. A link between sleep and brain plasticity is becoming clear in adults, as well.

Animal and human studies suggest that the quantity and quality of sleep have a profound impact on learning and memory. Research suggests that sleep helps learning and memory in two distinct ways. First, a sleep-deprived person cannot focus attention optimally and, therefore, cannot learn efficiently. Second, sleep itself has a role in the consolidation of memory, which is essential for learning new information.

Researchers now hypothesize that slow-wave sleep (SWS), that is deep, restorative sleep, also plays a significant role in declarative memory by processing and consolidating newly acquired information. REM sleep seems to plays a critical role in the consolidation of procedural memory. Other aspects of sleep also play a role: motor learning seems to depend on the amount of lighter stages of sleep, while certain types of visual learning seem to depend on the amount and timing of both deep, slow-wave sleep (SWS) and REM sleep.

Sleep is a necessary aspect of life and is essential to our health. It is recommended that we get eight hours of sleep every night.

The Harvard Women's Health Watch suggests six reasons to get enough sleep:

- **Learning and memory.** Sleep helps the brain to commit new information to memory.

- **Metabolism and weight.** Chronic sleep deprivation may cause weight gain by affecting the way our bodies process and store carbohydrates, and by altering levels of hormones that affect our appetite.

- **Safety.** A lack of sleep contributes to a greater tendency to fall asleep during the daytime. These lapses may cause falls or mistakes, such as medical errors, air traffic mishaps, and road accidents.

- **Mood.** Sleep loss may result in irritability, impatience, inability to concentrate, and moodiness. Too little sleep can also leave you too tired to do the things you like to do.

- **Cardiovascular health.** Serious sleep disorders have been linked to hypertension, increased stress hormone levels, and irregular heartbeat.

- **Disease.** Sleep deprivation alters immune function, including the activity of the body's killer cells. Keeping up with sleep may also help fight cancer.

GETTING YOUR EXERCISE

You probably already know that proper exercise can make you feel better, have more energy, and help you to live longer. The health benefits of regular exercise and physical activity are hard to ignore.

The benefits of exercise are present regardless of your age, sex, or physical ability, and they go far beyond just looking better in a swimsuit.

Exercise can help prevent excess weight gain or help maintain weight loss. When you engage in physical activity, you burn calories. The more intense the activity, the more calories you burn. Of course, even if you can't do an actual workout, you can get more active throughout the day in simple ways. Take the stairs instead of the elevator or take short strolls. Regular physical activity can help you prevent or manage a wide range of health problems and concerns, including stroke, metabolic syndrome, type 2 diabetes, depression, and certain types of cancer, arthritis, and falls.

Physical activity stimulates various brain chemicals that may leave you feeling happier and more relaxed. You may also feel better about your appearance and yourself when you exercise regularly, which can boost your confidence and improve your self-esteem. Regular physical activity can improve your muscle strength and boost your endurance. Exercise and physical activity deliver oxygen and nutrients to your tissues and help your cardiovascular system work more efficiently. And when your heart and lungs work more efficiently, you have more energy to perform your daily chores.

Regular physical activity can help you fall asleep faster and deepen your sleep. It can leave you feeling energized and looking better, which may have a positive effect on your sex life. It can lead to enhanced arousal for women. Men who exercise regularly are less likely to have problems with erectile dysfunction than are men who don't exercise.

Exercise and physical activity can also be a fun way to spend some time. It gives you a chance to unwind, enjoy the outdoors, or simply engage in activities that make you happy. Physical activity can also help you connect with family or friends in a fun social setting. Exercise and physical activity are a great way to feel better, gain health benefits, and have fun. Twenty minutes of physical activity every day is a good starting point. If you want to lose weight or meet specific fitness goals, you may need to exercise more. It's a good idea to check with your doctor before starting a new exercise program, especially if you have any health concerns.

Daily exercise reduces the risk of developing or dying from some of the leading causes of illness and death in the United States:

- Reduces the risk of dying prematurely.
- Reduces the risk of dying prematurely from heart disease.
- Reduces the risk of developing diabetes.
- Reduces the risk of developing high blood pressure.
- Helps reduce blood pressure in people who already have high blood pressure.
- Reduces the risk of developing colon cancer.
- Reduces the feelings of depression and anxiety.
- Helps control weight.
- Helps build and maintain healthy bones, muscles, and joints.
- Helps older adults become stronger and better able to move about without falling.
- Promotes psychological well-being.

Daily physical activity can help prevent heart disease and stroke by strengthening your heart muscle, lowering your blood pressure, raising your high-density lipoprotein (HDL) levels (good cholesterol) and lowering low-density lipoprotein (LDL) levels (bad cholesterol), improving blood flow, and increasing your heart's working capacity. Regular physical activity can reduce blood pressure in those with high blood pressure levels. Physical activity also reduces body fat, which is associated with high blood pressure. It can help to prevent and control Type 2 diabetes.

Physical activity helps to reduce body fat and build muscle mass. This improves the body's ability to use calories. When physical activity is combined with proper nutrition, it can help control weight and prevent obesity, which is a major risk factor for many diseases. By increasing muscle strength and endurance and improving flexibility and posture, regular exercise helps to prevent back pain. Regular weight-bearing exercise promotes bone formation and may prevent many forms of bone loss associated with aging.

Regular physical activity can improve your mood and the way you feel about yourself. Researchers have found that exercise is likely to reduce depression and anxiety and help you to better manage stress. Millions of Americans suffer from illnesses that can be prevented or improved through regular physical activity.

In our next chapter, we'll look at some exciting new ways to measure our wellness and body functions—tests that help us identify what's working and what's not, and treatments to correct our less-than-optimal results.

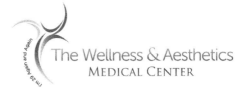
The Wellness & Aesthetics
MEDICAL CENTER

Chapter Nine

HEALTH ON THE CUTTING EDGE

The march of science is leading us toward exciting new areas of knowledge, including the kind of self-knowledge regarding our individual health that we could only dream of a few years ago. With the tools and tests available to us today, we can accurately pinpoint problems and correct them without the guesswork required before now.

Let's look at some of the options available to you today, not only in testing, but also in actually retraining your body systems to work more efficiently, based on those test results.

GENETIC TESTING

No two people are alike. Our genes determine much of how our bodies respond to our behaviors, external stimuli, and environment. Genetic testing is a proactive way for anyone ready to take control of his or her health and wellness through lifestyle modification.

For athletes, those who need help with weight management, and those with other lifestyle needs, genetic testing allows you to develop a custom, science-based solution based on individual genetic traits. Those include individual dietary preferences and behaviors and their effect on your metabolism as well as how your body responds to physical activity.

Analysis of more than 100 genetic markers allows a person to predict the effect of diet and exercise on specific areas of the body, including the brain, muscles, and pancreas. Testing allows us to gain more insight into how an individual processes fats, sugars and nutrients. Through combined genetic testing of a small saliva sample and an individual questionnaire, genetic testing removes the guesswork. That allows the provider to develop a more effective weight loss plan for you based on the following factors:

- **Diet:** Scientific studies demonstrate that certain nutrients turn specific genes on or off. We can now identify an individual's triggers.

- **Eating behaviors:** By identifying an individual's patterns, including snacking habits and timing of meals, we can help you develop a plan to modify your lifestyle in a way that will lead to weight loss.

- **Food reactions:** We all like certain foods but not always for taste. You can identify genetic markers that affect cravings for caffeine; sensitivity to the taste of salty, sweet and bitter foods and drinks; and lactose intolerance.

- **Nutritional needs:** The ability to feel full is partially dependent on the body's perception that it is receiving the nutrition it requires. Genetic testing allows you to determine the likelihood that you have an insufficient absorption of key nutrients, such as folate and vitamins.

- **Exercise:** Proper weight management lies somewhere between the foods we eat and the physical activity that converts it to energy. Genetic testing allows you to maximize your health and performance by predicting your response to exercise.

- **Ongoing weight management:** Genetic testing allows us to determine an individual's predisposition to obesity and to predict whether and how a person may regain weight following its loss. That allows for an ongoing plan that maximizes the potential for long-term success.

- **Metabolic health:** Obesity or even minimal weight gain can be a sign of metabolic imbalance. That imbalance can influence an individual's likelihood to develop health conditions, such as Type 2 diabetes and cardiovascular conditions, such as stroke and heart attacks.

NEUROINTEGRATION (NEUROFEEDBACK) TESTING AND TRAINING

What is neuroIntegration training?

At the Wellness and Aesthetics Medical Center, we use the Clear Mind Center NeuroIntegration System to optimize brain function. You cannot grow younger if your brain is not optimal.

Clear Mind Center has created a unique NeuroIntegration System, a groundbreaking approach in multi-sensory brainwave training. The photic technology informs the brain of the frequency it needs to learn and guides the brain into producing new, efficient brainwave states through EEG driven auditory and visual feedback. The system combines these technologies to achieve rapid improvement in mental and physical states, yielding powerful long-lasting results.

This multi-sensory approach interrupts ineffective mental patterns, lifting us out of habitual, non-productive thoughts. By balancing the brain and regulating the nervous system, new thought patterns are allowed to break through old filters responsible for causing a wide variety of disorders. NeuroIntegration Training has been proven to be a very powerful technique for improving brain functions.

Clear Mind Center's NeuroIntegration system works through a mechanism known as operant conditioning. When a part of the brain is operating at an abnormal frequency (too fast or too slow), the brain can learn to normalize the activity of that area.

How NeuroIntegration training works

The brain is a learning machine. If you signal the brain through photic stimulating lights, the brain will learn to make normal brainwave patterns through guided feedback. Continuous feedback retrains the brain to reduce abnormal activity and stay within normal ranges. Eventually, the brain learns how to stay within normal ranges without NeuroIntegration training, and is able to sustain normal activity independently. The mechanism is through reorganization of functional pathways in the brain.

Many breakdowns in health start with subtle changes in brain chemistry, which alter brainwaves in very specific ways. Brainwaves can be measured using electrodes similar to the ones used for an EKG. Research has found that a Quantitative EEG has high reliability, equal to such routine tests as an MRI and CAT scans.

A neuro-map is able to record patient brainwaves in real-time and offer a detailed visual report in minutes. In addition, a comprehensive neurological assessment plan with NeuroIntegration training protocols is provided to correct abnormal brainwave patterns found in the neuro-map. Research and clinical studies show that many cognitive conditions unresponsive to medication or psychotherapy can be resolved within 20–40 therapy sessions. At the other end of the spectrum, chronic disorders, such as anxiety, even if present over many years, can show improvement after just one treatment.

While genetics and birth complications can be contributing factors, research studies show that unresolved post-traumatic stress pushes the brain into patterns of chronic over-stimulation, gradually causing it to lose its ability to recover. Eventually, the traumatized brain must shut down for its own survival via depression, memory loss and other "protective" changes in brain function.

By normalizing brainwave patterns, your central nervous system learns how to self-regulate, directing you away from debilitating, painful, destructive disorders, into reclaiming your well-being.

Typically, clients experience a significant shift in awareness during their first session. Balancing the brain and calming the nervous system allows new neural patterns to form. Properly balanced rhythms result in optimal brainwave patterns. Our emotions are a reflection of the rhythms in our brains: excess beta can produce anxiety; too much frontal alpha could result in depression or ADD. Training brainwaves into efficient patterns allows the central nervous system to learn how to self-regulate, directing it away from debilitating, painful, destructive disorders into effortless processing and optimal functionality.

The features in the neuro-map report offer state-of-the-art technology, which present an in-depth analysis and guidance for NeuroIntegration Training. A professional and comprehensive report is provided. There at a glance, features provide the standard output of highly expensive research grade qEEG systems. In addition, areas of potential cognitive and emotional problems typically associated with specific map profiles are offered as a guide to validate patient's emotional and cognitive tracking.

The neuro-map recording takes approximately 12 minutes. Once the recording is complete, the data is uploaded to a neuro-map site for immediate processing. The final part of the neuro-map report offers suggested protocols based on the interpretation. These protocols are automated in the database and are available immediately after the report. These full-color visual reports offer an accurate and easy to use presentation. These reports offer a guide to the patient wellness. NeuroIntegration Training addresses problems of brain dis-regulation, which includes anxiety, depression, ADD/ADHD/OCD, chronic fatigue, fibromyalgia, head injuries, memory loss, migraines, PMS, post traumatic stress disorder, sleep disorders and performance enhancement.

PHYSIOAGE (AGE ANALYSIS) TESTING

At the Wellness and Aesthetics Center, we use PhysioAge for our biological age analysis. You cannot grow younger if you do not know how old you are. You are as old as your oldest organ. We can formulate a treatment program to optimize your oldest organs so they function better. Exercise, sleep, and healthy nutrition make all your organs and body functions better. There are other treatment programs to make your brain, lungs, heart, arteries, and skin younger and healthier.

....

How well are you aging?

- "The first step to aging well is knowing how well you are aging."
- Find out how fast you are aging.
- Identify your precursors to disease.
- Recognize your weakest body system.
- Receive a comprehensive, individualized health profile.

....

The PhysioAge Systems measures vital body systems to identify how well you are aging. While you may be 60 years old, your actual physiological (biological) age may be 70. Tracking physiological age over time provides a clear profile of your personal aging process, and can help your doctor determine which treatments to prescribe and when.

Built on solid science

Detail and precision are crucial differences that set PhysioAge Systems apart from other health tests. Their expert system is based on solid science: extensive clinical trials, scientific literature, and careful statistical analysis of primary data. Rather than using secondary clinical studies to calculate physiological age, they used their own in-depth, primary research to measure 120 attributes among 118 individuals. This study determined how biomarkers relate to each other, which enables a greater degree of statistical accuracy and a deeper understanding of the aging process. Biomarkers are levels in your body that can give some indication of status and risk. With unique in-house measurements, PhysioAge Systems gives you complete, clear, and precise results.

If you want to know how well each of your important body systems is aging, you should take the test. It can identify your weakest link and help you to do something about it before you develop a disease. Recognizing your body's unique strengths and weaknesses can help you achieve improved quality of life and sustained health. PhysioAge Systems provides a unique health profile that is tailored so that you can identify your current and future health status.

As an example, you may be 60 years old but have the arteries of a 75-year-old. Your doctor might want to address this risk by treating your cardiovascular system now, rather than waiting until you develop heart disease.

How does PhysioAge measure your health and aging?

PhysioAge measures your body's working age *using sophisticated biomarkers of aging.* Several painless, noninvasive tests are performed on you and a blood sample may be drawn. You will also take a 15-minute computerized brain function test. The results of these tests are submitted to a web-based reporting platform, which automatically generates a comprehensive report listing your physiological ages as well as easy-to-understand descriptions of up to 160 individual results.

THE FOLLOWING ARE THE SIX CORE BIOMARKERS OF AGING MEASURED BY PHYSIOAGE SYSTEMS:

- CardioAge—Arterial Stiffness Testing
  - Evaluates cardiovascular risk by measuring blood pressure at the heart to determine artery suppleness.

- CutoAge—Skin Elasticity Testing
  - Assesses the elasticity, firmness, and resistance of the skin with the same instrument used in numerous clinical trials for skin care products.

- PulmoAge—Lung Function Testing
  - Measures lung function, which is linked to many fatal diseases, not just lung disease.

- NeuroAge—Brain Function Testing
  - Assesses brain aging through a series of computerized tests focused on age-sensitive aspects of cognitive function.

- TelomerAge—Telomere Length Measurement

- □ Measures telomere lengths—caps at the ends of the chromosomes that shorten with every cell division—to indicate cell longevity.
- ImmunoAge—Immune Function Testing
    - □ Uses an advanced blood test to measure the health of your immune system.

Optional testing

- ImmunoAge
- TelomerAge

Other available tests

- Ultrasound CIMT (Carotid Intima-Media Thickness)
    - □ Detects sub-clinical atherosclerosis at the time when further progression can be prevented—long before your stress test is positive—without the radiation exposure of the heart scan.
- Bone Mineral Density Scan
    - □ Measures your propensity to develop osteoporosis using the latest GE LUNAR DEXA scanner.
- Body Composition Testing
    - □ Measures body fat and lean body mass using bioelectrical impedance.

TELOMERE & MICRONUTRIENT TESTING

At the Wellness and Aesthetics Medical Center, we use Spectrocell's telomere and micronutrient testing. It's important to know your levels before you begin nutrient supplementation. Supplementing with B-12 may be detrimental without the other B vitamins. Only supplementing with B-12 can deplete the other B vitamins.

The Telomere test is the window to your true cellular age. This advanced test measures the length of your telomeres (the end caps of your DNA). Studies have shown a direct link to telomere length, cardiovascular health and the aging process.

Overwhelming scientific evidence confirms that vitamin deficiencies are associated with disease processes and the overall condition of one's health. Vitamin, mineral, and antioxidant deficiencies have been shown to suppress immune function and to contribute to chronic degenerative processes, such as arthritis, cancer, Alzheimer's, cardiovascular disease, and diabetes.

The Micronutrient tests measure how micronutrients are actually functioning within your white blood cells. These tests allow nutritional assessment of a broad variety of clinical conditions, including arthritis, cancer, cardiovascular risk, diabetes, various immunological disorders, metabolic disorders, and micronutrient deficiencies.

Before micronutrient testing, many diagnosis and risk assessments were based on clinical observation and measurements of static levels of certain nutrients in serum. Static serum levels are not always representative indicators for assessing cell metabolism and utilization. Micronutrient testing offers a unique means to scientifically assess the intracellular requirements of micronutrients that play an important role in overall health and wellness of a person. The tests measure the biochemical function of vitamins, minerals, amino acids, and antioxidants, providing a powerful clinical assessment tool.

The functional intracellular status of micronutrients involved in cell metabolism is evaluated by manipulation of the individual micronutrients in the media, followed by mitogenic stimulation and measurement of DNA synthesis. The ability of cells to resist damage caused by free radicals and other forms of oxidative stress should be measured also. Due to the considerable number of cellular antioxidants with extensive interactions, redundancies, repair and recharging capabilities, measuring total function is the most accurate and clinically useful way to assess a person's capacity to resist oxidative damage.

With all of these cutting-edge scientific tools to help us establish where you are on the age spectrum, we're now able to offer individualized therapies that can take years off of your actual age, and optimize your wellness. But we realize that feeling younger is only a piece of the big picture, even though it's a key piece. In order to get you back to 29 again, another big piece is how you look—to others, and to yourself when you look in the mirror. Let's explore some of the amazing ways that your youthful looks can be brought back.

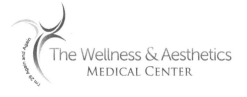
Chapter Ten

LOOKING YOUNGER

SKIN CARE & OPTIMIZATION

So far, we have worked on our insides, but as we've observed, growing younger must include looking younger. At the Wellness and Aesthetics Medical Center, we use multiple media to help you look younger. Among these are laser therapy with Sciton, body sculpting using Pure Lipo, stem cells usage, and PRP (Platelet Rich Plasma) to stimulate stem cell and growth factors activation for joints, muscles, neck, face, and male and female genitalia.

My Five Step Skin Rejuvenation Program is designed to take years off your skin and help you look younger. It involves **Skin Detoxification, Volume Optimization, Bio-identical Hormone Optimization, Nutritional (Vitamin, Mineral and Herbs) Optimization and Ongoing Skin Care**. Unlike my Five Step Wellness Program, this is for everyone.

Step 1. Skin Detoxification

Skin detoxification removes free radicals, toxins, and heavy metals from the body. It helps you lose weight and improves your immune system. It decreases premature aging and gives you softer, smoother, younger, brilliant skin. The Sciton Laser is one of the primary instruments of detox at the Wellness and Aesthetics Medical Center. See www.LookBeautifulAgain.com

Step 2. Volume Optimization

As we age, we loose volume in our skin. Replacing the volume loss is essential to looking younger. At the Wellness and Aesthetics Medical Center we use dermal fillers, Pure Lipo fat, stem cells, and Plasma Rich Platelet (PRP) as in our Vampire Facelift and Cell Assisted facial fat transfer.

Step 3. Bio-identical Hormone Optimization

Optimizing our hormones helps with collagen formation, bone and muscle. These are required to maintain a youthful look. They help against wrinkle formation, age spots and decreases the need for detoxification.

Step 4. Nutrition (Vitamin, Minerals and Herbs)

We use oral, topical, intramuscular and intravenous nutrition to optimize the body and skin. Once the skin is ablated with our sciton, the skin absorbs the nutrition much more readily. The dead skin is removed and a healthy layer of skin appears. PRP induces the stem cells in the areas placed to become younger and healthier.

Step 5. Ongoing Skin Care

At the Wellness and Aesthetics Medical Center our goal is a younger, healthier you. Looking younger is essential to our program. After the first four steps we continue to treat the skin on a periodic frequency with nutraceuticals, laser treatments, fillers, and PRP.

Chemical peels & fillers

Fillers are injectable gel that adds volume and hydration to your skin, smoothing away unsightly wrinkles and folds. Each filler composition is unique. Treatment is nonsurgical, meaning there's minimal recovery time.

Radiesse is an FDA-approved injectable filler used to restore facial fullness. Radiesse works with the body to promote the natural growth of collagen, filling in furrows and lines between layers of skin. The procedure takes less than an hour, and medication is available to deal with slight discomfort at the points of injection. Results are immediate, lasting nine to 15 months. Many people are highly pleased with the combination of Radiesee and Botox, together rewinding years off of faces.

Restylane is a safe, effective, nonsurgical gel injection that enhances lips by restoring volume. With a treatment time of just 30 minutes and little to no downtime, you can achieve voluptuous, youthful lips with no interruption of normal life. The result is immediate, producing long-lasting and safe natural enhancement. Restylane® can help you look younger and healthier.

Juvedurm is a smooth, injectable gel that adds volume and hydration to your skin, smoothing away unsightly wrinkles and folds. Its composition is unique, providing a high concentration of cross-linked hyaluronic acid for long-lasting, most-natural results. Treatment is nonsurgical, meaning there's minimal recovery time.

Belotero is an injectable filler that combines with water to plump and fill in wrinkles. It is made of hyaluronic acid. It works instantly and ameliorates the lines and wrinkles in the face. It also works on the nasolabial folds and smokers lines of the lips. At the Wellness and Aesthetics Medical Center, it is the filler of choice.

Sunspots, vascular and pigmented lesions

Over time, our skin loses its resistance to the sun's harmful UV rays. This susceptibility can be seen in age spots. Photo rejuvenation is a fast, painless way to dramatically reduce their appearance and treat sun damage, using specially tuned lasers and filters to spur the replacement of damaged skin. The procedure is quick, with no downtime afterwards.

Benign vascular lesions are a common problem for many. Unsightly veins ranging from telangiectasias (small widened blood vessels on the skin) or spider veins, to deeper vascular lesions can now be treated effectively with laser therapy.

Photo Rejuvenation

Increasingly, more patients demand fast, effective treatments aimed at restoring their skins' natural beauty, to eliminate blemishes, and give them a healthier, fresher look.

With a wide array of interchangeable filters, a laser can treat a variety of skin lesions such as dyschromia, hyperpigmentation, melasma, ephelides, warts, scars, striae, port wine stains, hemangiomas, telangiectasias, rosacea, angiomas, hair removal, and much more.

Botox

Botox is often called the "facelift in a bottle." It's a simple, non-surgical procedure that relaxes the muscles responsible for wrinkles. Nearly 90 percent of people surveyed rate their improvement moderate to better one month after treatment. Botox treatments are quick—usually 10–15 minutes will keep the facial muscles relaxed for up to

4–6 months. The procedure is simple and minimally invasive, and results are dramatic and easy to see.

Xeomin

At the Wellness and Aesthetics Medical Center, Xeomin is the muscle relaxer we use. We have used both Xeomin and Botox. The Xeomin have been far superior to Botox. It's easier to use, less expensive, and offers better patient outcome.

Laser treatment for vascular, skin lesions, acne, and scars

The **Micro Laser Peel** is for individuals who want to be refreshed without missing a beat. It is especially suited to treat aged skin associated with an active lifestyle. Many people call it the "weekend" skin peel, yielding instant long-term results without time off, discomfort, or post-treatment care. Using a precise computer-guided laser and variable treatment depth, the skin is revitalized while maximizing tonal evenness.

Skin Resurfacing is for those of us looking for a more gradual skin rejuvenation plan. It is aimed toward long-term results, involving a steady, personalized treatment regimen to renew and recondition skin over time. With a variety of procedures and the promotion of healthy skin habits, this option ensures that your skin is renewed, and thereafter preserved.

Do you have visible veins that draw unwanted attention to your legs? Spider veins affect millions of men and women. These veins appear as red, blue, or purple lightning-shaped lines and are most often found on the thighs, calves, or buttocks. The unsightly appearance of telangiectasias, spider veins, and deeper vascular legions makes many people uncomfortable in their own skin. If you suffer from spider veins, there is a safe and effective treatment available for you. **Laser vein treatment** is effective on all skin types, using an array of specialized filters to target vascular blemishes quickly, accurately, and in maximum comfort.

Acne is a common condition usually associated with teenagers, but may also affect adults. A few recurring pimples constitutes mild acne, whereas tens or hundreds of inflamed areas signifies severe acne. Unfortunately, it has been shown that a person cannot typically treat acne effectively on his or her own. Since acne has been proven to be unrelated to such lifestyle factors as diet or hygiene, changes in these lifestyle factors are ineffective. Living with acne can lead to anxiety, antisocial behavior, and scars that can last a lifetime. But long-term relief from acne is possible with laser therapy. Treatment is traditionally topical or with antibodies, but laser therapy has proven to be a faster and more precise way to remedy acne and acne scars.

Laser therapy is a process whereby a laser technician will heat the sebaceous glands in the dermis (top layer) of the skin. This reduces oil production, leading to noticeable reductions in active acne in two to four weeks. Results of this acne treatment have been documented to last up to six months.

LASER HAIR REDUCTION

Tweezing, shaving, and waxing are costly and time-consuming. With laser hair reduction, unwanted hair can be removed quickly and easily from anywhere on the body. Using new highly specialized technology, hair is removed effectively and with the fewest number of treatments. Laser technology can remove hair from just about any area of the body, but most common locations include the upper lip, the chin, legs, armpits, and bikini line. During laser hair reduction, technicians use heated light to damage the deepest portions of the hair follicles without damaging the surrounding skin. This process hinders future hair growth. Four days prior to laser hair reduction, patients should refrain from waxing, tweezing, or tanning the treatment area. Laser hair reduction has no recovery period, so patients can resume daily activities as soon as they leave the office.

PROFRACTIONAL LASER THERAPY

ProFractional is a quick and comfortable laser procedure, with little to no downtime, used to improve the overall appearance of your skin. ProFractional uses a laser microbeam to treat thousands of pinpoint areas of your skin. And because only a fraction of the skin is directly treated with the laser, healing time is quick and downtime is short. The zones of untreated skin invigorate the body's natural healing process, and the treated areas stimulate production of new collagen, plumping up the skin and smoothing out wrinkles, lines, scars, and other irregularities.

PROFRACTIONAL CAN BE USED TO IMPROVE A WIDE VARIETY OF SKIN CONDITIONS, BUT IS USED MOST FOR:

- Wrinkles and fine lines
- Post-traumatic scars
- Acne scars
- Age spots
- Sun spots
- Freckles, aging, and sun-damaged skin

Facial rejuvenation with stem cells

Cell-assisted autologous fat transfer is a procedure in which a patient's own body fat is used to augment sunken or thin regions of the face in order to add volume where it is desired. PRP (Platelet-Rich Plasma) is combined with the fat and stem cells prior to facial insertion. This procedure is a safe and scientifically proven process where fat cells are harvested and redistributed to the face to eliminate wrinkles and facial droops.

THIS TYPE OF FAT TRANSFER HAS SUCH APPLICATIONS AS:

- Filling in forehead wrinkles and laugh lines
- Filling sunken areas under the eyes
- Cheek or chin augmentation
- Smoothing lines in the face
- Improve facial symmetry
- Lip augmentation

With cell-assisted autologous fat-transfer, a majority of the transferred fat remains in its place permanently, which means long-lasting results. There is also very little risk for post-procedure complications.

Even though it may sound complex, autologous fat transfer is a simple procedure, requiring just four steps.

1. Excess fat from abdomen, buttocks, thighs, or jowls is removed.
2. Fat cells are isolated and cleansed.
3. Stem cells are extracted from the fat and mixed with PRP.
4. The fat cells are then injected into the specified facial areas, along with the PRP and stem cells.

Vampire facelift

The Vampire Facelift provides a way to help restore shape, improve tone and texture, and rejuvenate new and younger tissue by activating stem cells with PRP. It uses a filler like Juvederm (hyaluronic acid) in a very specific way to sculpt a younger, natural-appearing face. Then, PRP is extracted from the patient's own blood with the use of a centrifuge. The PRP is activated to release at least eight growth factors. These growth factors work to increase collagen and new blood flow. With the use of a tiny needle, the PRP is inserted into the appropriate area of the face. The PRP activates the multipotent stem cells, which then develop into new collagen, blood vessels, and fatty tissue to improve the skin.

Platelet-Rich Plasma (PRP)

Another application involving Platelet Rich Plasma (PRP) therapy is an injection treatment that stimulates the growth of new tissue using blood plasma with concentrated platelets. These platelets contain bioactive proteins, which are vital to initiating growth and accelerating tissue repair. This new treatment can help regenerate tendon or ligament tears common with sports injuries and heal arthritic degenerative joints.

As in the Vampire Facelift, in order to create PRP, the patient's own blood sample is placed in a centrifuge that separates the platelets from the other components. The concentrated platelet-rich plasma is then injected into the damaged area, stimulating the tendon or ligament, and significantly facilitating the body's natural tendency to heal itself. PRP activates stem cells with the help of the growth factors released from it. A new muscle tissue begins to develop as a result of the injection, and as it matures it begins to shrink, tightening and strengthening the tendons and ligaments of the damaged area.

The PRP treatment will heal the muscle tissue with minimal or no scarring, and it alleviates further degeneration as it builds new tissues. Because the patient's own blood is used, there is no risk of a transmissible infection and a very low risk of allergic reaction. The need for surgery or any kind of long-term medication is reduced greatly with PRP therapy.

PRP injections can provide help for all areas of the body, including the face; **cervical, thoracic, and lumbar spine; wrists, elbows, shoulders, hips, knees, and ankles; as well as tendons and ligaments**. The treatment will also help patients with injuries such as tennis elbow, carpal tunnel syndrome, scoliosis, ACL tears, shin splints, rotator cuff tears, plantar faciitis, and iliotibial band syndrome.

The treatment has received enhanced media coverage in recent months thanks to New York Yankees star Alex Rodriguez, who received plasma-rich platelet injections following a recommendation from Los Angeles Lakers star Kobe Bryant. Rodriguez had undergone surgery on his right knee and also had problems with his left shoulder, but was dissatisfied with the recovery process. Bryant's positive experience with the PRP treatment led Rodriguez to travel to Germany and receive the therapy.

Laser Skintyte & wrinkle reduction

Over time, our skin loses its resilience. Where our skin was once smooth, wrinkles have formed like cracks in a dry riverbed. Wrinkle reduction does exactly what it says—reduces those unsightly cracks. SkinTyte is a formidable weapon in fight against aging and gravity. It uses deep dermal heating to reverse the sagginess of aged skin. Using a specially tuned laser that targets the collagen layer in skin, those wrinkles are broken down, returning your skin to the elasticity of its youth. This procedure is commonly applied to droopiness under the eyes, jowl and neck, brow lines, and nasolabial folds—quickly, painlessly, and without any interruption of normal life. With a personalized treatment plan typically consisting of three to four treatments, in little time your skin will lose the sag, appearing tighter and many years younger.

Cellulite and Stretch Marks Reduction

The Wellness and Aesthetics Medical Center uses the Synergie Aesthetic Massage System and Sciton's SkinTyte for cellulite treatment. We have had tremendous success with this system.

Cellulite or stretch marks are common in both men and women:

- 80–90 percent of post-pubertal females suffer from cellulite.
- Cellulite is not a substance and cannot be surgically eliminated.
- It is caused by inconsistent rigidity of collagen columns just below skin's surface.
- Appearance of cellulite is not correlated to obesity—even thin women deal with cellulite.

Until recently, there has been no reliable treatment for cellulite. Even weight reduction is not a cure for cellulite. The Synergie Aesthetic Massage System (AMS) can reduce cellulite. The FDA-approved Synergie machine employs a revolutionary vacuum massage technology that has been proven to enhance skin smoothness. Synergie has been the cellulite solution for countless happy patients.

The skin being stretched beyond its full capacity causes stretch marks. Stretch marks most often occur around the breasts or the stomach during puberty, pregnancy, or rapid weight gain. Unfortunately, these scars do not diminish with breast reduction, termination of pregnancy, weight reduction, or time.

Sciton's SkinTyte laser treatment can also reduce or eliminate these ugly marks, as it also reduces cellulite. It heats the skin and tightens the tissues beneath the surface and triggers the body's natural healing process.

Features of a SkinTyte treatment include:

- No creams or lotions (which are unproven in stretch mark treatment)
- Greatly decreased visibility of stretch marks
- No recovery time, so you can resume your daily activities right away

With all of these wonderful new tools and procedures at your disposal, there's no excuse for looking older than you want to.

HAIR REGROW

You cannot look younger without a full head of hair. At the Wellness and Aesthetics Medical Center, we address hair loss with nutrition optimization, toxic metal detoxification, and bio-identical hormonal optimization. We also use a low-level laser cap and PRP scalp injections (as in Vampire Hair Regrow).

We have been having tremendous success with these therapies.

Visit http://www.twaamc.com or www.sciton.com to see before and after photos.

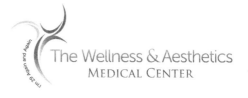

Chapter Eleven

FUNCTIONING YOUNGER

*J*ames is a 72-year-old widower, a retired accountant who lives in Houston, Texas. He has been in a four-month relationship, but was concerned because he had not been able to have an erection in 12 years. He was treated for prostate cancer 11 years ago. His health care provider recommended he get a penile prosthesis.

James and his girlfriend came to the Wellness and Aesthetics Medical Center to see me six months ago. He had a three-hour evaluation that included in-clinic testing and a two-hour consultation with me. We discussed the benefits of testosterone. His girlfriend was very interested when she learned that testosterone affects the heart more than any other organ in the body and the brain second. They were both shocked that testosterone can be used in both men and women. They were surprised to learn that testosterone protects against heart disease, sharpens memory and cognitive function, helps sleep, improves work performance, decreases stress, and protects against Alzheimer's disease and dementia. They were very surprised that normal testosterone does not cause prostate cancer.

In the clinic, we were able to give him an 85 percent erection that lasted one hour and fifteen minutes. He also had his testosterone checked. He was given a six-month supply of testosterone pellets to optimize his testosterone to that of a much younger man. His girlfriend also made an appointment to have her hormones optimized and now gets pellet therapy.

When we saw them again at their recent evaluation, they had gotten married. They felt invigorated, were enjoying a healthy sex life, and both stated they "felt 20 years younger."

We are almost at our destination. Our journey included stops at Feeling Younger, Growing Younger, and Looking Younger. We are now ready to Function Younger. At the Wellness and Aesthetics Medical Center, we make this journey with our friends every day.

ERECTILE DYSFUNCTION (MALE & FEMALE ORGASMIC THERAPY)

Erectile dysfunction (impotence) is the inability to get an erection, a problem keeping an erection firm enough for sex, and/or a reduced sexual desire. When you suffer erectile dysfunction on an ongoing basis, it can impact negatively on your self-confidence, cause stress, and can create relationship problems between your partner and you.

An erection is an emotional event that begins in the brain. Physical and/or mental stimulation cause nerves in the brain to send chemical messages to nerves in the penis, telling the penile blood vessels to relax so that blood can flow freely into the penis. Once in the penis, high pressure traps the blood within both *corpora cavernous*. This causes the penis to expand and sustain an erection. Erection is reversed when the inflow of blood is stopped and opening outflow channels open, allowing the penis to become soft.

Who suffers from erectile dysfunction (ED)? Erectile dysfunction is three times more common in men who have diabetes and is most often caused by poor long-term blood sugar control, which damages nerves and blood vessels. Erectile dysfunction can be linked to other conditions common in men with diabetes, such as high blood pressure and coronary artery disease. ED in diabetes is associated with vascular and neural factors. Hyperglycemia (increased glucose in blood) is believed to give rise to these microvascular changes. ED in diabetes is strongly correlated with glucose control, duration of the disease, and diabetic complications. The incidence increases with increasing age, duration of diabetes, and deteriorating metabolic control, and is higher in individuals with Type 2 diabetes than in those with Type 1. ED in men with diabetes often affects their quality of life; as patients are often reluctant to come forward with their symptoms, they miss the opportunity to correct their ED.

Male sexual arousal is an intricate process that involves the brain, hormones, emotions, nerves, sexual arousal, muscles, and blood vessels. Erectile dysfunction can result from a problem with any of these. In most cases, erectile dysfunction is caused by something physical.

Specific causes of erectile dysfunction (other than diabetes):

- Metabolic syndrome (a condition involving increased blood pressure), high insulin levels, body fat around the waist, and high cholesterol
- Obesity, inflammation
- Low testosterone
- Tobacco, alcoholism, and other drug abuse
- Heart disease, high blood pressure, neurological disease
- Peyronie's disease (development of scar tissue inside the penis)
- Parkinson's disease, multiple sclerosis disease
- Surgeries or injuries that affect the pelvic area or spinal cord

- Medications such as antidepressants, antihistamines, and medications to treat high blood pressure, pain, or prostate cancer.

- Emotional or psychological distress

- Depression, anxiety, or other mental health conditions

- Problems due to money, stress, fatigue, relationships, work, chronic fatigue syndrome, or fibromyalgia

A medical history and a physical exam are all that's needed before a doctor is ready to recommend a treatment.

Common tests for possible underlying problems may include:

- Blood tests to check for signs of heart disease, diabetes, low testosterone, hormone levels, and other health problems

- Simple urine tests to look for signs of diabetes and other underlying health conditions

- Ultrasound to check blood flow to your penis. It involves using a wand-like device (transducer) held over the blood vessels that supply the penis. This test is sometimes done in combination with an injection of medications into the penis to determine if blood flow increases normally.

- Overnight erection test that involves wrapping special tape around your penis before you go to bed. If the tape is separated in the morning, your penis was erect at some time during the night without you being able to feel it. This indicates the cause of your erectile dysfunction is most likely psychological and not physical.

- Nerve test to check neuronal integrity

Treatment is often more successful when a man involves his partner. Getting the right treatments for any health problems that could be causing or worsening your erectile dysfunction should be your first step. For years, the principal treatments have been either medical/drugs or surgical. Today, regenerative medicine offers you a new approach: Stem cells from your own fat or bone marrow, or platelet-rich plasma (PRP) from your own blood, can be used to repair the problem, rather than putting a band-aid on the problem with drugs such as Viagra or Cialis.

ICP

ICP (intracavenous pharmacotherapy), combined with testosterone optimization and suction therapy, can be very successful in treating Erectile Dysfunction (ED) and Premature Ejaculation (PE). The penis is a muscle, which can atrophy because of decreased usage. With the combination therapy, the penis can be exercised on a daily basis. This allows the muscle to increase in size. The blood flow and nervous system improves and erection is improved. Adding PRP and stem cells speeds up the process.

A Priapus shot with PRP is also effective in reducing ED. The PRP activates the muscles, arteries, and nerves in the penis. The stem cells are also activated by the PRP in the penis. When combined with ICP, dilator, high-dose arginine, and testosterone, the results are significantly improved.

Women's Orgasm (O-Shot)

The *Journal of the American Medical Association* reports that sexual dysfunction, often considered worse in women than in men, can lead to a lowered sense of well-being that negatively affects the relationships with our sex partners and can contribute to the disintegration of the family. Sexual disorders not only take the fun out of sex, but better sex also leads to greater energy, more creativity, increased confidence, less depression, and improved overall health.

....

Here are some of the common areas of sexual dysfunction experienced by many women:

- **Low desire:** Also known as Hypoactive Sexual Desire Disorder (HSDD), this is not counted as a disorder unless it disrupts the woman's life. According to the National Institute of Health, as many as 26.7 percent of premenopausal women and 52.4 percent of naturally menopausal women experience HSDD. About 12.5 percent of women who enter surgically induced menopause experience HSDD.

- **Female Sexual Arousal Disorder:** Affecting about one in 20 women, this usually — but not always — accompanies HSDD. Women who experience this may want to have sex but have much difficulty finding the pleasure of arousal.

- **Female Orgasmic Disorder:** Again, around one in 20 women can become aroused but have much difficulty with orgasm. This can become so frustrating that some women who experience orgasmic disorder may avoid sex altogether.

- **Dyspareunia:** This condition causes up to 10 percent of women to suffer real physical pain with sex. This is pain not caused by decreased lubrication or vaginal spasm.

....

Up to 50 percent, or 75 million, American women report experiencing some level of physical sexual dysfunction. Many more who never report their sexual disorders may be affected. As a result, many learn to tolerate less than optimal sexual activity rather than activating the female orgasm system.

Why do so many women suffer in silence? Research shows that only about 14 percent of women EVER talk to ANY of their physicians about sex. With up to half of women experiencing a sexual disorder, why do only about one in 10 ever talk to their physicians about sex?

According to *Practice Bulletin in Obstetrics and Gynecology*, one reason may be that research has led to few proven treatment options. To date, treatment generally is limited to hormone replacement therapy, in the form of vaginal estrogen or topical testosterone. Even with hormone therapies, results are short-term.

Only 14 percent of doctors ever discuss sexual problems with women. If the woman receives hormone replacement therapy, the only other known solution, per the official recommendation of the American College of Obstetrics and Gynecology, appears to be psychosocial therapies. Under the circumstances, both physician and patient would be discouraged from discussing a problem for which there is no proven solution—so the doctor just doesn't ask. There's no doubt that sex education/counseling helps sexual performance and results, but if the woman's body does not respond as it should even with proper knowledge, then the woman continues to suffer. That explains why up to 75 million women in the United States alone continue to suffer mentally and physically from sexual problems.

But new therapies, and familiar ones used in new ways, have appeared and are working miracles for women suffering sexual dysfunction. For several years, blood-derived growth factors have been used to regenerate the face. Biopsy studies published in highly regarded medical journals, such as *Advances in Skin & Wound Care* and *Journal of Drugs in Dermatology*, demonstrate that when platelet-rich plasma (PRP) is injected, stem cells multiply and grow new younger tissue. In the same way that PRP regenerates the skin of the face, it appears PRP regenerates healthy vaginal tissue. Relying on this same technology, the O-Shot® procedure works by using PRP to stimulate stem cells to grow healthier vaginal tissue.

The whole procedure for processing the blood and injecting the growth factors takes less than 10 minutes in the doctor's office. There is no magic shot to take the place of emotional, hormonal, relationship, and general health.

The O-Shot® procedure begins with a simple blood draw. Using a proprietary technique, the growth factors in platelet-rich plasma (PRP) are extracted from that blood sample and injected into an area near the clitoris and into a the area of the upper vagina that is most important for the sexual response, the O-Spot. Because these areas have been numbed with a local anesthetic cream, patients experience little or no discomfort during the procedure.

The "O" Shot helps with the following:

- Urinary Incontinence

- Vaginal Lubrication

- Pain with intercourse

- Orgasm

ADRENAL FATIGUE

Adrenal fatigue is produced when your adrenal glands cannot adequately meet the demands of stress. The adrenal glands mobilize your body's responses to every kind of stress (physical, emotional, or psychological) through hormones that regulate energy production and storage, immune function, heart rate, muscle tone, and other processes that enable you to cope with the stress. Whatever emotional crisis (divorce, death of a loved one, financial problems, a physical crisis such as major surgery, or any type of severe repeated or constant stress in your life) you have, your adrenals have to respond to the stress and maintain homeostasis. During adrenal fatigue, your adrenal glands function but not well enough to maintain optimal homeostasis, because their output of regulatory hormones has been diminished. Over-stimulation of your adrenals can be caused either by a very intense single stress, or by chronic or repeated stresses that have a cumulative effect.

You may be experiencing adrenal fatigue if you have the following symptoms:

- You feel tired for no reason.
- You have trouble getting up in the morning, even when you go to bed at a reasonable hour.
- You become very emotional.
- You are feeling rundown or overwhelmed.
- You have difficulty bouncing back from stress or illness.
- You crave salty and sweet snacks.
- You feel more awake, alert, and energetic after 6 p.m. than you do all day.

PELLET THERAPY

For men and women, aging can come with unwelcome fluctuations in hormones. Many synthetic oral or transdermal hormone replacement therapies are available, but they also can have less-than-desirable side effects, including mood swings.

At the Wellness and Aesthetics Medical Center, we use pellets from Biote. Their pellets use hormones derived from natural plant sources to replicate the body's normal hormonal levels. BIuTE® **Medical Hormone Pellet Therapy**, provides sustained hormone levels throughout the day, for up to six months without any "roller coaster" effect. The hormones are dispersed by blood flow. Someone who exercises a lot will use up pellets faster than one who is sedentary.

Biologically identical to estradiol and testosterone found in humans, pellet therapy can provide the benefits of hormone replacement for up to six months without the side effects experienced by some using synthetic hormones. Smaller than a grain of rice, the all-natural pellet is placed in the fatty tissue under the skin, where it provides consistent release of small hormone doses.

Pellet therapy has been clinically shown to be effective against a variety of symptoms in women as their estrogen levels decline. It can help maintain bone density, moderate sleeplessness, and alleviate migraine or menstrual headaches. For women experiencing deterioration in sexual well-being, pellet therapy can restore the sex drive, enhance sexual response, and decrease vaginal dryness. In women who suffer from incontinence, pellet therapy can reduce urinary urgency and frequency.

Men as young as 35 may notice a seemingly unexplainable fatigue, decline in mental clarity or sexual dysfunctions, such as loss of libido, or challenges in achieving or maintaining an erection. Almost all men should have their testosterone levels tested starting around age 35. Pellet therapy can help restore testosterone to levels near those of normally functioning testicles.

For many individuals using pellet therapy, they may see improved skin tone and hair texture. For some, muscle mass and bone density will build up as fat melts away. That may lead to increased strength, coordination, and physical performance.

Studied for more than 80 years, pellet therapy is used on five continents. For those concerned about sustained use of pellet therapy, clinical data supports its long-term effectiveness and safety. The pellets are totally biodegradable, leaving no residue under the skin.

Pellet therapy also supports those adhering to ethical vegetarian and vegan lifestyles. The estrogen and testosterone used in the pellets are extracted from natural plant sources and compounded according to strict federal guidelines.

FITNESS & EXERCISE

We talked in an earlier chapter about the importance of regular exercise, but it bears repeating: There are 1,440 minutes in a day. We can schedule 30 of those minutes to exercise. Regular exercise is a critical part of staying healthy. People who are active live longer and feel better than those who aren't active. Exercise can help you maintain a healthy weight. It can delay or prevent diabetes, some cancers, and heart problems. Exercise burns fat, builds muscle, lowers cholesterol, eases stress and anxiety, and lets us sleep restfully. Regular exercise can help boost energy, maintain your independence, and manage symptoms of illness or pain. Exercise can even reverse some of the symptoms of aging. And not only is exercise good for your body, it's also good for your mind, mood, and memory.

Exercise increases nitrous oxide. This improves vascular endothelial function, which, in turn, decreases risk of heart disease and strokes. According to William Osler, "A man is as old as his blood vessels." Our vascular system is our superhighway that transports micronutrients, oxygen, fuel, and cells to wherever they are needed. The system also transports substances to the liver to be detoxified or created. If this highway becomes blocked or congested, we could have tissue death and loss of life. Aerobic or endurance exercise

(AE) imposes a volume overload on the cardiovascular system with increased VO2 (oxygen consumption), heart rate, cardiac output, stroke volume, reduced systemic vascular resistance, decreased diastolic BP, and increased A-VO2.

The kind of exercise you do, and at what levels of intensity, is dictated by your current level of physical fitness. Jogging, swimming, biking, and other forms of continual movement should be done at specific levels of submaximal and maximal aerobic capacity (MAC) or estimated heart rate for age and level of exercise (MHR; 60–90 percent of 220 – age). One of the best techniques is aerobic interval training, which consists of short periods, ranging from 20 seconds to two minutes, of "burst" aerobic training of varying intensities, depending on one's present level of exercise conditioning (i.e., 80–90 percent MAC, then 50 percent MAC for 1–3 times that interval). This more closely mimics the natural activities we evolved to perform and benefit from, and strings together several periods of intense and semi-intense activity into a single, longer exercise period that still burns calories and builds endurance.

Resistance training (RT) exerts both a volume and pressure overload state with little change in heart rate, cardiac output, or stroke volume. Systolic BP initially increases, but over time there is little change in systolic or diastolic BP. RT either increases or does not change VO2.

Weight lifting, modified properly, will encourage optimal muscle physiology and release of hormones, mediators, and interleukins. Lift the heaviest weight possible 12 times to get the muscle burn, then decrease the weight with each subsequent set. Keep increasing the number of times that weight is lifted. This maximizes post-exercise oxygen consumption, depletes glycogen, and increases the production of lactic acid to achieve all the muscle-, hormone-, cytokine-, and interleukin-stimulating effects that lead to the health benefits of exercise.

The optimal ratio of resistance to interval aerobic training should be 2:1. For example, during a 60-minute workout, you would perform 40 minutes of resistance training and 20 minutes of interval aerobics (40/20 minutes), with the aerobics coming after the resistance training. This should be done at least four days per week. You should rotate upper and lower body muscles, core (exercises designed to improve abdominal and back strength while increasing flexibility; these exercises are important for the core—abdomen and lower back—which is often neglected), flexibility, and agility.

Drinking plenty of water while working out is imperative. (If you get thirsty during the workout, you have waited too long to drink.) You must drink water before beginning to exercise, at set intervals during exercise, and afterwards. Your water should be of high quality (alkaline) and not from plastic containers, due to the risk of certain chemical compounds, such as Polychlorinated biphenyls (PCBs), that get into the water from the plastic.

Ten minutes after starting your workout, begin consuming an energy drink such as orange juice, dextrose, or raw honey with water, d-ribose, carnitine, glutamine, and whey protein, and other supplements to provide ATP and energy as well as nutritional substrates to maximize exercise performance and increase muscle strength and performance as well as lean muscle mass.

Exercising in the morning after a 12-hour fast is best. An empty stomach optimizes fat burning, IL-10 (Interleukin 10, decreases inflammation, increases serum testosterone and growth hormone and fat metabolism, regulates glucose, reduces weight, increases lean muscle mass, optimizes fuel metabolism, and reduces the risk of MI and stroke), and myokine surges. This results in an increase in muscle strength, bulk, tone, and contour, as well as weight loss and improved energy level, focus, and concentration during the day.

Mastering proper breathing techniques will ensure ample oxygenation for the muscle performance, as well as prompt the removal of carbon dioxide. Consumption of a carbohydrate supplement immediately after exercise improves insulin action and synthesizes muscle glycogen significantly faster than when the same amount of carbohydrate is consumed two hours post-exercise. The timing of whole protein may not be as crucial as the timing of specific amino acid supplements and anabolism. Most studies suggest that consuming free amino acids immediately prior to exercise or within 10 minutes of the initiation of exercise is more effective to increase muscle protein accretion, compared to consumption after exercise.

Whey protein supplies glutathione precursors (cysteine, glutamine), is anabolic, with an increase in muscle mass, and reduces oxidative stress and inflammation. The ingredients in whey help maximize ATP (adenosine triphosphate) production, improve muscle performance, increase muscle mass, and reduce muscle fatigue.

....

Dr. Houston's 60-minute exercise regimen

Into a 32-ounce bottle add the following:

- 6 ounces of fresh orange juice

- 1 Tablespoon of organic raw honey (30% glucose, 30% fructose, 30% other sugars)

- 30-40 grams of whey protein powder

- Amino acid blend: 6.6 grams of leucine, lysine, isoleucine, valine, threonine, histadine, cystine, phenylalanine, methionine, tyrosine, tryptophan

- 10 grams of D-ribose powder (provides immediate ATP production for energy, improved mitochondrial function, cardiovascular support, reduction in Reactive Oxygen Species (ROS), inhibition of the breakdown of adenine nucleotides during hypoxia/ischemia and cellular protection with increased reduced glutathione levels)

- 2 grams of carnitine tartrate powder (improves beta-oxidation in skeletal and cardiac muscle by transport of fatty acids longer than C-12, which provides energy to all muscles. Carnitine is also an excellent antioxidant and reduces exercise-induced oxidative stress, decreases fatigue, enhances muscle performance and endurance)

- 2 grams of glutamine powder (increases muscle growth and glutathione induces gastrointestinal repair, improves immune function and exercise performance)

- 2 grams of taurine powder (decreases muscle soreness and muscle damage during and following high intensity exercise that is additive to BCCA)

- 2 grams of arginine powder with 1000 mg citrulene (increases nitric oxide, increases exogenous carbohydrate oxidation and decreases the oxygen cost of exercise)

- Cordyceps 3000 mg standardized (an adaptogen that increases MVO2, RBC delivery, coronary vasodilation, Increase ATP / O2 utilization by 15%, improve performance and stamina. 3000 mg po. Standardized to 0.14 % adenosine / 5% mannitol)

- Rhodiola 300 mg standardized (an adaptogen that decrease exercise HR, reduce NE and EPI, increase serotonin and beta-endorphins, and reduces arrhythmias. Improves performance (mental and physical), decrease fatigue 20% 300 mg po. Standardized to 5% rosavin / 1% salidroside)

□ 2 grams of arginine powder with 1 gram citrulene phyto-supplements before exercise: Have additive effects in combination

....

Within 30 minutes post-exercise, Dr. Houston recommends BCAA (branch chain amino acids—leucine, isoleucine, valine). This increases muscle mass, muscle protein synthesis, and anabolism via mRNA translation, reduces muscle damage, accelerates recovery and provides important amino acids (especially leucine); 3000 mg at ratio 4:1:1, and a balanced meal with CHO/ Protein 4/1 to 1/1, good fats, fruits and vegetables; a proprietary high-dose vitamin supplement, 5 caps BID (VS) proprietary high-dose EFA (Omega 3 FA), with tocopherols; 6 caps BID (EFA) Resveratrol: 250 mg per day Creatine: 5 grams. You need minimum of 5 grams protein/15 minutes of exercise. Also, prior exercise increases anabolic effects of nutrients to muscles, and improves vasodilation.

BENEFITS OF EXERCISE:

- Reduces risk of MI, recurrent MI, angina, CHF
- Reduces cardiac arrhythmias
- Improves cardiac function, ejection fraction, cardiac index, and cardiac output
- Improves coronary blood flow and reserve, oxygen consumption, aerobic capacity, LVEDV (Left Ventricle End-Diastolic Volume)
- Improves congestive heart failure both systolic and diastolic
- Reduce CVA (Cardiovascular Accident)

- Increases eNOS (endothelial nitric oxide synthase) and NO (nitric Oxide)

- Improves endothelial function and vasodilation

- Lowers blood pressure and heart rate

- Improves heart rate variability (HRV), decreases sympathetic nervous system (SNS), and increases parasympathetic activity (PNS)

- Reduces total cholesterol, triglycerides, LDL, VLDL, and increases HDL

- Lowers blood glucose, decreases risk of diabetes and improves diabetes

- Increases androgens/testosterone, growth hormone, estradiol and progesterone

- Improves insulin sensitivity and levels

- Improves conversion of T4 (inactive thyroid hormone) to T3 (active thyroid hormone)

- Decreases cortisol, catecholamines, and aldosterone

- Improves immune function and decreases infection, except with overtraining

- Increases muscle mass and decreases sarcopenia (resistance exercise)

- Improves memory and focus and reduces risk of Alzheimer's disease and dementia

- Improves skin tone and elasticity and decreases wrinkles

- Improves depression, stress, and anxiety, and overall psychological well-being (neurotransmitters)

- Improves sleep and sleep quality and insomnia
- Reduces risk of certain cancers, such as colon, breast, and prostate
- Decreases risk of gallstones and peptic ulcer disease
- Increases telomerase, slows telomere attrition rate and slows aging
- Decreases oxidative stress with proper training
- Reduces inflammation
- Decreases fatigue and improves energy levels
- Decreases osteoporosis
- Improved quality of life

Exercise and optimal sleep are the most fundamental issues in growing younger. Without adequate amount of each, we cannot grow younger. The third leg in growing younger is nutritional optimization, which we will discuss in the next chapter.

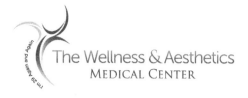

The Wellness & Aesthetics
MEDICAL CENTER

Chapter Twelve

NUTRITIONAL OPTIMIZATION

N utrition is the means of providing the materials necessary to support life. Poor nutrition destroys life. High-quality (optimal) nutrition supports a healthy lifestyle. The body is an incredible machine. Given proper nutrition, the body can eradicate illness and optimize our health. Minerals, vitamins, and enzymes are the tools the body needs to make or breakdown any and all body processes. Without them you cannot make a hormone, neurotransmitter, protein, cell, or enzyme.

The GI tract readily absorbs organic nutrition. Inorganic nutrition is poorly absorbed. Healthy fats, natural sugars, and protein should be consumed. HFCS (High Fructose Corn Syrup), artificial sweeteners, diet drinks, energy drinks, coffee, tobacco, and alcohol should be avoided. Foods rich in antioxidants should be consumed.

Fat helps your body to absorb fat-soluble vitamins, such as A, D, E, and K, and contributes to gall bladder health. Fats also help you lose weight by giving you a sense of fullness and adding texture to your meals. Other benefits of consuming fats include turning off the insulin pump, decreasing triglyceride levels, increasing metabolism, protecting muscle membranes, and protecting your brain from memory loss.

189

Coconut oil consists of medium chain triglycerides (MCT). It is converted to energy in the liver without the insulin spike. It improves cardiac and thyroid functions, increases metabolism, promotes lean body mass, and supports a healthy immune system.

Vegetables are nutrient dense, low-glycemic carbs, and high in essential fiber that helps promote a healthy bowel. The average American eats less than two servings of fruits and vegetables per day—far below the 7–9 servings that we need.

Soluble fiber dissolves in water, slows the breakdown of complex carbs, and helps to reduce blood sugar. When taken in large quantities, it can help reduce cholesterol. It is found in grains, vegetables, fruits, and legumes. Insoluble fiber doesn't dissolve in water and is not absorbed or digested. It reduces hunger, keeps the GI system clean, and promotes healthy bowel movements. It is found in brown rice, whole-wheat products, seeds, vegetable and fruit skins, and legumes.

You should eat more anti-inflammatory foods such as herbs (ginger, rosemary, turmeric, oregano, cayenne, cloves, nutmeg, feverfew, and boswellia). Teas contain catechins, which reduce inflammation. White tea is highest in catechins, followed by green, then black tea. Chocolate also contains catechins as well as polyphenols, another antioxidant. Wine, red wine in particular, has powerful antioxidants and has been shown to have anti- inflammatory capabilities. Anti-oxidant supplements include carotenoids, vitamins C and E, bioflavinoids, glutathione, alpha-lipoic acid, selenium, and phytonutrients. Immune-supporting supplements include vitamins A, C, and D, magnesium, zinc, copper, molybdenum, CoQ10, and arginine. Energy-supporting supplements include B vitamins, biotin, inositol, iron, magnesium, vanadium, L-carnitine, chromium, and CoQ10. Probiotics should be taken every day and increased on stressful days or when taking antibiotics.

Nutrition for the brain includes: fish oil, extra virgin olive oil, canola oil, herbs that replenish neurotransmitters and remove beta-amyloid (such as turmeric, basil, black pepper, sage, mint, lemon, and rosemary). Also supportive of brain health are vitamins A, E, and B6, acetyl-L-carnitine, alpha lipoic acid, phosphatidylserine, CoQ10, zinc, selenium, magnesium, ginkgo biloba, lecithin, green tea, and Omega-3 fatty acids.

Optimizing T3 (the active thyroid) is essential for energy, immune function, and brain and cardiac function. It is also imperative for your cells ability to perform their functions.

Foods with low glycemic index and loads are essential. Only eat food that runs, jumps, hops, flies, swims, crawls, hangs from trees, or grows on a vine or root. Even with everything above, you still need nutritional supplementation, such as organic multivitamins, minerals, and enzymes.

OPTIMAL SLEEP

Are you an early riser or a night owl? Schedule your sleep time. Prior to bed, decrease stimulation, turn off your cell phone and TV, decrease liquid intake, exercise, avoid alcohol, take your medication, and resolve any stressors/family issues. Prepare your bedroom for maximum relaxation (light, scent, temperature ventilation, color, bed, and decluttering). Prepare yourself with a bath or shower, appropriate clothing, and footwear. Getting into bed, you may want to meditate, read a light book, or cuddle with someone. You need a minimum of six to seven hours of sleep per night — optimally, eight hours.

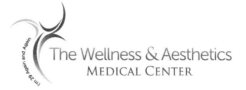

The Wellness & Aesthetics
MEDICAL CENTER

Resources and References

Additional resources can be found at:
www.twaamc.com/l-arginine.html

Anon. *Better Fighting Through Chemistry? The Role of FDA Regulation in Crafting the Warrior of the Future.*

Bearn, Alexander G. (1976). "Structural Determinants of Disease and Their Contribution to Clinical and Scientific Progress." SIBA Foundation Symposiums *44*, pp. 25–40.

Caffeine and Sports Performance. Vanderbilt.edu.

CDC/NCHS. (2012). Health, United States, 2012, Figure 10. Data from the National Health and Nutrition Examination Survey.

Christian, Henry A. (1947). *The Principles and Practice of Medicine.* 16th Edition. New York: D. Appleton-Century, p. 582.

Food and Drug Law: Final Paper. Harvard.edu. March 8, 2004.

Classen, J. Barthelow. (1996). "Childhood Immunisation and Diabetes Mellitus." *New Zealand M.J., 109* (May 24, 1996): 195.

Coulter, H. L., and Fisher, Barbara Loe. (1991). *DPT: A Shot in the Dark*. Garden City Park, NY: Avery Publishers.

Easmon, C.S.F., and Jeljaszewicz, J. (1983). *Medical Microbiology*, Volume 2. *Immunization Against Bacterial Diseases*. London and New York: Academic Press.

Ehrengut, Wolfgang. (1990). "Central Nervous System Sequelae of Immunization Against Measles, Mumps, Rubella and Polio-myelitis." *Acta Paediatrica Japonica 32*: 8–11.

Furman, B. L., Wardlaw, A. C., and Stevenson, L. Q. (1981). "Bordetella Pertussis-Induced Hyperinsulinemia Without Marked Hypoglycemia: A Paradox Explained." *British Journal of Experimental Pathology 62*: 504–511.

Gold, Daniel H., and T.A. Weingeist, T. A. (1990). *The Eye in Systemic Disease*. Philadelphia: Lippincott.

Lavi, Sasson, et al. (1990). "Administration of Measles, Mumps and Rubella Vaccine (Live) to Egg-Allergic Children." *Journal of the AMA 263* (2) (January 12, 1990): 269–271.

Menser, Margaret, et al. (1978). "Rubella Infection and Diabetes Mellitus." *Lancet* (January 14, 1978): 57–60.

Munoz, J. J., and Bergman, R. K. (1977). *Bordetella Pertussis*. New York and Basel: Marcel Dekker.

Numazaki, Kei, et al. (1989). "Infection of Cultured Human Fetal Pancreatic Islet Cells by Rubella Virus." *Am. J. Clinical Pathology 91*: 446–451.

Pollock, T. M., and Morris, Jean. (1983). "A 7-Year Survey of Disorders Attributed to Vaccination in North West Thames Region." *Lancet* (April 2, 1983): 753-757.

Rayfield, E. J., et al. (1986). "Rubella Virus-Induced Diabetes in the Hamster." *Diabetes 35* (December 1986): 1278–1281.

Sekura, Ronald D., Moss, Joel, and Vaughan, Martha. (1985). *Pertussis Toxin.* New York and London: Academic Press.

Smith, Pamela Wartian, *What You Must Know About Vitamins, Minerals, Herbs & More: Choosing the Nutrients That Are Right for You.* Square One Publishers, 2007.

Somers, Suzanne. *I'm Too Young for This!: The Natural Hormone Solution to Enjoy Perimenopause.* Harmony, 2013.

Stites, Daniel P., Stobo, John D., Fudenberg, H. Hugh, and Wells, Vivian J. (1984). *Basic and Clinical Immunology.* 5th Edition. Los Altos, CA: Lange; 152ff.

Tingle, Aubrey J., et al. (1985). "Postpartum Rubella Immunization: Association with Development of Prolonged Arthritis, Neurological Sequelae, and Chronic Rubella Viremia." *J. Infectious Diseases 152* (3) (September, 1985): 606–612.

Yesalis, Charles. (2007). *Anabolic Steroids in Sport and Exercise*. Champaign, IL: Human Kinetics.

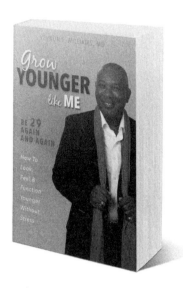

How can you use this book?

MOTIVATE

EDUCATE

THANK

INSPIRE

PROMOTE

CONNECT

Why have a custom version of *Grow Younger Like Me?*

- Build personal bonds with customers, prospects, employees, donors, and key constituencies
- Develop a long-lasting reminder of your event, milestone, or celebration
- Provide a keepsake that inspires change in behavior and change in lives
- Deliver the ultimate "thank you" gift that remains on coffee tables and bookshelves
- Generate the "wow" factor

Books are thoughtful gifts that provide a genuine sentiment that other promotional items cannot express. They promote employee discussions and interaction, reinforce an event's meaning or location, and they make a lasting impression. Use your book to say "Thank You" and show people that you care.

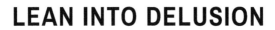

LEAN INTO DELUSION